Medical Microbiology Practical Record Book

Authors

Dr. Gurjeet Singh
PhD, DIPC, MBA, PGDHA
Professor
Department of Microbiology
M.M. Institute of Medical Sciences and Research,
Mullana, Ambala, Haryana

Dr. Raksha
PhD, MBA, PGDHA
Professor
Department of Microbiology
M.M. Institute of Medical Sciences and Research,
Mullana, Ambala, Haryana

Peepee Publishers and Distributors Private Limited®

Medical Microbiology Practical Record Book

Published by
Pawaninder P. Vij and Anupam Vij

Peepee Publishers and Distributors Private Limited
Head Office: 160, Shakti Vihar, Pitam Pura, Delhi-110 034 (India)

Correspondence Address:
7/31, First Floor, Ansari Road, Daryaganj
New Delhi-110 002 (India)
Ph: 41512412, 9811156083
e-mail: peepee160@yahoo.co.in
e-mail: peepee160@gmail.com
www.peepeepub.com
join us on facebook.com/pp.publishers

First Edition: 2025

ISBN: 978-81-9720-722-8

Dedication

This Medical Microbiology Practical Record book
is dedicated to our beloved twins daughters

Jasleen Kaur (Eshika)
and
Jasveen Kaur (Eshita)

"Burn worldly love, rub the ashes and make ink of it,
Make the heart the pen, the intellect the writer, write that which has no end or limit."

Guru Nanak

"Teachers open the door, but you must enter by yourself"

Chinese Proverb

"A person who never made a mistake never tried anything new"

Albert Einstein

"Learning is never done without errors and defeat"

Vladimir Lenin

FOREWORD

Writing the foreword for the Medical Microbiology Practical Record Book, authored by Dr. Gurjeet Singh and Dr. Raksha, gives me immense joy. The writers have made an effort to finish this practical record book, which covers all practical needed for students to acquire the skills and knowledge they need. The wording is quite clear and basic, making it very easy for the pupils to understand the purpose of each experiment.

This practical record book includes practical exercises accompanied by a list of learning objectives that assist students in understanding the experiment and gaining knowledge and skills related to the experiment. There is plenty of space to write notes in the practical record book as well. As needed, students can utilize this space to jot down detailed information pertaining to their expertise.

It is a gratifying fulfillment of a much desired need, and the authors are deserving of all recognition and appreciation for having tried to fill it in a credible and significant way. With the help of this medical microbiology practical record book, I hope that the students will have great success.

Dr. Hariom Sharan
Professor and Head
Department of Microbiology
Autonomous State Medical College,
Firozabad, Uttar Pradesh.

FOREWORD

It gives immense pleasure to write the foreword for Dr. Gurjeet Singh and Dr. Raksha's Medical Microbiology Practical Record Book, intended for undergraduate and graduate students, brings me great joy. Teachers worked hard to create this book.

This book has all the practical material needed to learn medical microbiology, along with enough of space for students to write down any pertinent details.

The development of new abilities and other significant tasks necessary for the academic program are documented in this book. It is a gratifying satisfaction of a much desired need that the author has made an effort to fill in a credible and significant way, and for that, they are well deserving of recognition and gratitude.

Dr. Yogendra Pratap Mathuria
Professor
Microbiology Department
All India Institute of Medical Sciences,
Rishikesh, Dehradun, Uttarakhand

FOREWORD

[illegible]

FOREWORD

I am delighted to contribute the foreword for the Microbiology Practical Record and Logbook, which was co-authored by Dr. Gurjeet Singh and Dr. Raksha. In order to adequately prepare students, the writers have made every effort to finish this practical record book which covering all practical abilities. One of the trickiest medical microbiology topics are made entertaining and simple with the help of this practical record book, which provided simplified explanations of complex concepts. Students find it quite easy to comprehend the purpose of each experiment due to the clear and simple language.

This practical record book incorporates self-directed learning where students are required to illustrate the life cycles of important parasites in order to increase their confidence.

My best wishes are extended to both authors on the successful publication of their valuable practical record book. This practical record book will undoubtedly improve students' abilities and knowledge while also improving their learning.

Dr. Rajesh Bareja
Professor and Head
Department of Microbiology
World College of Medical Sciences and Research,
Jhajjar, Haryana

PREFACE

It gives us great pleasure to offer the "Medical Microbiology Practical Record Book" with sincere gratitude. This practical record book is created for students of medical microbiology. It included all of the material and practical requirements that students would need. Students will have plenty of space in this practical record book to write down their experiments and other pertinent data. It is written in an approachable, transparent, and basic style to get students ready to study about medical microbiology.

Every experiment of this practical record book contains laboratory practices step-by-step with practical diagnostics microbiology.

The aim of this practical record book is to provide practical guide for students. This practical record book was outlined using compressed knowledge to make one of the most difficult subjects of medical microbiology as one of the most interesting and simplest subjects. The simple and easy to understand language have been used to make it very easy for the average students to understand the content of each experiment.

This medical microbiology practical record book has 41 practical's. Each practical has learning objectives so that students may understand the importance of the experiment and gain knowledge and skills following the experiments.

Our profound gratitude is extended to M/s. Peepee Publisher and Distributors Private Limited for their assistance, endurance, and interest in the release of this practical record book on medical microbiology.

Dr. Gurjeet Singh

Dr. Raksha

Medical Microbiology Practical Record Book

Department of Microbiology

Affix your recent passport size photograph here

Student's Personal Details

Name of Student : ____________________

Father's Name: ____________________

Name of College / University : ____________________

____

Date of admission: ____________________

Roll No . ____________________

Registration No. (University Registration No.) ____________________

Permanent Address :

____

____

____

____

E-mail ID ____________________

Mobile No. ____________________

Certificate

This is to certify that

Mr./ Ms. ____has attended all the experiments entered in this practical record book and that his/her progress has been satisfactory.

Semester/Year	Remark	Signature of in- charge & Date
I	Completed ☐ Not completed ☐	
II	Completed ☐ Not completed ☐	
III	Completed ☐ Not completed ☐	

I/c Practical Programme
Signature & Stamp

Professor & Head
Signature & Stamp

Seal

INDEX

SYLLABUS FOR MEDICAL MICROBIOLOGY

GENERAL MICROBIOLOGY

Topic	Must Know	Desirable to Know
History & Microscopy	• Definitions of Medical Microbiology, Pathogen Commensal, Symbiotic. • Contribution of : - Louis Pasture - Robert Koch - Joseph Lister - Paul Ehrlich • Names of scientists who discovered common bacteria • Importance of Microbiology	
Morphology of bacteria I	• Difference between Prokaryotes & Eukaryotes • Microscopy – Basic principle and applications of all microscopes • Classification of staining techniques • Gram's stain and ZN stain in detail (with examples) • Negative staining, Impregnation method • Albert's stain • Special stains	
Morphology II	• Morphology of Bacteria - different shape and size • Different unit of measurement • Bacterial cell anatomy in detail • Bacterial Spore • Bacterial flagella • Bacterial capsule • Bacterial pili	
Physiology of bacteria	• Bacterial cell division, Generation time, Bacterial growth curve • Bacterial growth requirements • Redox potential (Eh)	Bacterial Metabolism
Sterilization	• Definitions of Sterilization, disinfection, asepsis, antiseptics • Need of Sterilization / Disinfection in various fields – Medical, Food & Pharma Industry • Physical methods of Sterilization Sunlight, Heat (dry & moist heat), Filtration, Radiation in details	
Disinfection	• Characteristics of ideal chemical disinfectant • Factors influencing potency of a disinfectant • Disinfectants like Aldehydes , Alcohols, Halogens, Oxidising agents, Salts, SAA, Gases, Dyes (Concentration, Mode of action and uses only)	Testing of Disinfectants
Culture Media	• Types of Media and their uses	Composition of Media

Culture Methods	• Types of aerobic culture methods and their uses • Types of anaerobic culture methods and their uses • Mc Intosh Filde's Jar – Functioning and uses	
Identification of bacteria	Morphology of bacteria (Gram stain), Motility Biochemical tests (Principle and examples)	Morphology of Bacterial Colony Biochemical tests (Procedure) Typing Method Pathogenicity tests
Antimicrobial therapy	Mode of action of antimicrobial agents Antibiotic Sensitivity tests : Kirby Bauer disc diffusion Importance of making an antibiotic Policy Strict Adherences to antibiotic Policy	Antibiotic Sensitivity tests: Stokes Disc diffusion E-test Dilution test

Bacterial Genetics	Basic structure of Bacterial DNA
	Definitions of Gene, Codon, Nonsense codons
	Extrachromosomal elements – Plasmids, Episomes, Transposons
	• Difference between Phenotypic & Genotypic variation (Mutation)
	• Genetic Variation (Mutation)
	• Gene transfer (Transformation, Transduction, Lysogenic conversion, Conjugation)
	  • Differences between Mutational & Transferable drug resistance
	  • Mechanism of drug resistance
		• Synthesis of Polypeptide (Transcription and translation)
		• Genetic Engineering
		• DNA Probes
		• PCR
		• Gene therapy

Bio- medical waste disposal	• Definition of Biomedical waste • Classification, disposal and treatment as per categories • Importance of segregation	
Universal Safety Precautions & health care associated infections	• Universal safety precautions • Hand Hygiene • Definition of Hospital acquired infection. • Sources, types, prevention and control of health care associated infections	
Normal microbial flora of human body	Introduction – Various sites, types & role	
Infection Host parasite relationship	• Definitions of Saprophytes, Parasitic, Commensals, Pathogen, Opportunistic Pathogens, Pathogenicity, Virulence • Types of infection, Routes of transmission • Sources of Infection • Difference between Exotoxins & Endotoxins • Types of Infectious diseases Localised, Generalised, Endemic, Epidemic, Pandemic	Factors Predisposing to Microbial Pathogenicity

SYSTEMIC BACTERIOLOGY
Format of study -
A: Classification
B: Morphology
C: Culture Characteristics
D: Biochemical reactions
E: Antigens
F: Pathogenesis & diseases caused in detail
G: Laboratory diagnosis
H: Prevention & control
I: Special identification tests

Topic	Must Know Subtopics	Desirable to Know
Staphylococci	A,B,C,E,F,G,H,I	D
Streptococci	A,B,C,E,F,G,H,I	D
Other streptococci and Pneumococci	A,B,C,E,F,G,H,I	D
Neisseria	A,B,C,E,F,G,H,I	D
Corynebacterium diptheriae	A,B,C,E,F,G,H,I	D
Mycobacterium tuberculosis	A,B,C,E,F,G,H,I	D
Atypical mycobacteria/ Non-tuberculous mycobacteria (NTM)	Name of the Species Names of the diseases caused Special tests for identification Brief outline of lab diagnosis	
Mycobacterium leprae	A,B,C,E,F,G,H,I	D
Bacillus	Name of the Species Names of the diseases caused Special tests for identification Brief outline of lab diagnosis	
Method of anaerobiasis & Non-sporing anaerobes	Method of anaerobiasis Nonsporing anaerobes (Name of the Species, Names of the diseases caused Special tests for identification, Brief outline of lab diagnosis)	
Clostridium – I	A,B,C,E,F,G,H,I	D
Clostridium – II	A,B,C,E,F,G,H,I	D
Enterobacteriacae – I (Escherichia coli.)	A,B,C,E,F,G,H,I	D
Enterobacteriacae – II Proteus & Klebsiella	A,B,C,E,F,G,H,I	D
Enterobacteriacae –III Salmonella	A,B,C,E,F,G,H,I	D
Shigella	A,B,C,E,F,G,H,I	D
Vibrio	A,B,C,E,F,G,H,I	D

Campylobacter & Helicobacter	Name of the Species Names of the diseases caused Special tests for identification Brief outline of lab diagnosis	
Pseudomonas	A,B,C,E,F,G,H,I	D
Other GNB I (Yersinia, Pasteurella, Francisella, Bordetella)	Name of the Species Names of the diseases caused Special tests for identification Brief outline of lab diagnosis	
Other GNB II (Haemophilus, Brucella)	Name of the Species Names of the diseases caused Special tests for identification Brief outline of lab diagnosis	
Miscellaneous Bacteria (Newer Bacteria)	Name of the Species Names of the diseases caused Special tests for identification Brief outline of lab diagnosis	
Spirochaete - I	A,B,C,E,F,G,H,I	D
Spirochaete - II	A,B,C,E,F,G,H,I	D
Actinomycete and Nocardia	A,B,C,E,F,G,H,I	D
Rickettsia	Name of the Species Names of the diseases caused Special tests for identification Brief outline of lab diagnosis	
Chlamydia	Name of the Species Names of the diseases caused Special tests for identification Brief outline of lab diagnosis	
Mycoplasma	Name of the Species Names of the diseases caused Special tests for identification Brief outline of lab diagnosis	
Bacteriology of water, Air & Milk	Bacteriology of Air Bacteriological Examination of Air Acceptable limit of Air pollution	Bacterial flora in water Water Borne Pathogens Bacteriological Examination of water Milk Borne diseases Bacteriological Examination of milk

MYCOLOGY

Topic	Must Know Subtopics	Desirable to Know
Introduction to mycology	• Introduction to Mycology • Difference between fungus & Bacteria • Classification of fungi with examples • Reproduction & Sporulation • Lab diagnosis of mycosis • Classification of Fungal diseases	
Agents of superficial mycosis (Dermatophytes)	• Superficial Mycosis a. Enumerate agents b. Predisposing factors c. Lab diagnosis (Outline)	Colony characteristics of dermatophytes
Subcutaneous mycosis & Candida	• Subcutaneous Mycosis & Candida in detail a. Enumerate agents b. Predisposing factors c. Lab diagnosis (Outline)	
Systemic mycosis & opportunistic fungal infections & Pneumocystis carinii	• Systemic & Opportunistic Mycosis a. Enumerate agents b. Predisposing factors c. Candida, Cryptococcus in detail d. Mucor, Aspergillus	Histoplasma, Pneumocystis carinii

VIROLOGY [n=16]

Topic No	Topic	Must Know Subtopics	Desirable to Know
01	General virology – I	• Morphology of Viruses • Replication of viruses	• Chemical properties of viruses • Susceptibility to physical and chemical agents • Viral Haemagglutinin
02	General virology – II	• Cultivation of Viruses ,Viral assays • Outline of diagnosis of viral diseases	
03	Virus-host interactions	• Inclusion Bodies • Routes of transmission of viral infections • Interferons • Immunity in viral diseases	• Host responses to virus infections

04	Viral vaccines and antiviral agents	• Commonly used viral vaccines a. Types and Schedule • List of antiviral agents.	Mode of preparation Chemoprophylaxis & Chemotherapy of viral diseases
05	Pox viruses Bacteriophage	• Morphology • Names of poxviruses and diseases caused • Bacteriophage [Basic structure and Significance]	Cultivation
06	Herpes simplex & Varicella zoster CMV, EBV	• Morphology • Classification • HSV (Infections caused and Lab diagnosis) • Varicella – Zoster (Infections caused and Lab diagnosis)	• EBV (Infections caused and Lab diagnosis) • CMV (Infections caused and Lab diagnosis)
07	Other DNA viruses (Papova, Adeno,)	Basic morphology, diseases caused	
08	Orthomyxoviruses	• Differences between Orthomyxo and paramyxo virus • Influenza Virus a. Morphology b. Antigenic classification and structure c. Antigenic shift and Antigenic drift d. Pathogenesis and lab diagnosis	Influenza Virus - Antigenic classification and structure - Prophylaxis Bird flu
09	Paramyxoviruses	• Morphology • Measles virus and Mump Virus	• Para-influenza virus • RSV
10	Picornaviruses	• Classification • Polio virus in detail • Differences between killed and live vaccines • Eradication and Prophylaxis of Polio virus	• Coxsackie viruses • Rhino virus
11	Hepatitis viruses	• HAV (Pathogenesis and Lab diagnosis) • HBV (Morphology, Mode of transmission, Clinical features, Lab diagnosis) • HCV (Morphology, Mode of transmission, Clinical features, Lab diagnosis) • HDV & HEV (Pathogenesis & Lab diagnosis)	

12	Arboviruses	• Classification , Names of Arboviruses and diseases caused • Dengue Virus in detail	JE yellow fever KED
13	Rhabdoviruses	• Morphology • Pathogenesis and Lab diagnosis • Prophylaxis	
14	Retro Viruses – HIV	• Morphology • Resistance • Modes of Transmission • Pathogenesis • Opportunistic infections and malignancies • Lab diagnosis in detail • Prevention • PEP	• Viral genes & antigens • ART
15	Miscellaneous viruses	• Viruses (Only names) causing gastroenteritis • Viruses causing viral hemorrhagic fevers (only names) • Slow virus diseases (Only names)	
16	Oncogenic viruses	Papilloma Virus Only names of oncogenic viruses and malignancies caused	

IMMUNOLOGY

Topic	Must Know Subtopics	Desirable to Know
Immunity	• Innate Immunity – Types, Factors influencing innate immunity, Mechanisms • Acquire Immunity - a. Active Immunity b. Passive Immunity • Combined immunization • Adoptive immunity • Local Immunity • Herd Immunity	
Antigen	• Types of Antigens • Factors affecting antigenicity	• Super antigens

Antibody	• Properties of antibodies • Structure of Immunoglobulin classes • IgG, IgM, IgA, IgD, IgE a) Basic structure, function & distribution	-IgG, IgM, IgA, IgD, IgE -Molecular weight, -Sedimentation coefficient -Abnormal Immunoglobulins
Antigen-antibody reactions	• Types of Ag – Ab reactions, precipitation, Agglutination, CFT, Neutralization, Opsonisation, Immunoflourescence, ELISA Immunochromatography (Principle, Types & uses only)	
Complement	• Components of complement • Classical Pathway • Alternative Pathway • Biological effects of complement • Deficiencies of complement	• Regulation of complement activation • Biosynthesis of Complement • Quantitation of complement
Structure & function of immune system	• Central Lymphoid Organs • Peripheral Lymphoid Organs • Cells of Lymphoreticular System • HLA • Differences between T & B cells	• Lymphocytic recirculation
Immune response	• Humoral Immune Response a) Primary and secondary responses b) Production of Antibodies c) Monoclonal antibodies d) Factors influencing antibody production • Cell mediated Immune Response a) Cytokines & Lymphokines – Types & functions only	• Cell mediated Immune Response a) Detection of CMI • Immunological tolerance
Hypersensitivity	• Definition & Classification • Type 1 Reaction • Differences between Immediate & delayed hypersensitivity • Type 2, 3 & 4 Reactions	
Autoimmunity	• Definition & Mechanisms • Classification with examples	
Immunodeficiency diseases		• Primary Immunodeficiency Syndromes & • Secondary Immunodeficiency (Only classification)

• Transplantation & Tumor immunity	• Types of Transplants • Allograft reaction • Histocompatibility Antigens • Histocompatibility Testing • Graft - Versus – Host reaction • Tumor antigens	• Immunosurveillance • Immune response to malignancy • Immunotherapy of cancer

- **PARASITOLOGY**

Topic No	Topic	Must Know Subtopics	Desirable to Know
01	Introduction to parasitology	• Classification of Parasites • Type of Parasites • Hosts (Definitive & Intermediate) • Host – Parasitic relationship • Sources of Infection • Lab diagnosis in general	
02	E.Histolytica	• Morphology • Life cycle • Pathogenesis & Complications • Lab diagnosis & treatment • Non Pathogenic amoebae • Free living amoebae	
3	Giardia, Trichomonas	• Giardia lamblia (Morphology, life Cycle, Pathogenesis, Lab diagnosis & treatment) • Trichomonas vaginalis (Morphology Pathogenesis, Lab diagnosis & treatment	
4	Malaria	Life Cycle, Morphology, Pathogenecity & Lab diagnosis, prevention	
5	Haemoflagellates	• Leishmania (Classification, diseases caused) L. donovani in details Morphology, Life cycle, Pathogenesis, Lab diagnosis	Trypanosoma brucci & Trypanosoma cruzi in details
6	Miscellaneous protozoa	• Toxoplasma (Morphology life Cycle, Pathogenesis, Lab diagnosis)	Cryptosporidium, Isospora B.coli
7	Cestodes	Taenia & Echinococcus (Morphology life Cycle, Pathogenesity, Lab diagnosis)	Brief mention about othercestodes
8	Trematodes	• Schistosomes a. Names & diseases caused	Morphology, Life Cycle, Pathogenicity & Lab diagnosis Fasciola hepatica

			Parognimus westermani
9	Nematodes (Intestinal)	• Ancylostoma duodenale, Ascaris lumbricoides, Enterobius vermicularis, Trichuris trichura (in details)	S. stercoralis
10	Tissue Nematodes I	Wuchereria bancrofti (in details) Trichinella spiralis	
11	Tissue Nematodes II & Stool concentration techniques	• Dracunculus medinensis (in details) • stool concentration techniques • Name of parasites in stool • Names of parasites affecting CNS • Names of parasites affecting liver • Names of parasites entering through skin • Bile stained eggs & Eggs which float in saturated salt solution & those which do not	

APPLIED MICROBIOLOGY

Topic No	Topic
	Only Causative agents & Brief Outline of Lab diagnosis in
1	• Gastrointestinal infections
2	• Upper respiratory tract infection (URTI)
3	• Lower respiratory tract infection (LRTI)
4	• Urinary tract infection (UTI)
5	• Central nervous system (CNS) infections
6	• Wound and Pyogenic infections
7	• Pyrexia of unknown origin / fever (PUO/PUF) and infections
8	• Sexually transmitted diseases (STDs)

EXPECTED ATTITUDE OF STUDENTS IN MICROBIOLOGY

1. The student will be regular, sincere, punctual and courteous.
2. Wearing an apron is compulsory.
3. The student will follow all the rules laid down by the department
4. The student will be regular in his/her studies.
5. The student will handle all the material /equipment supplied with care
6. The student will participate actively in seminars and projects.
7. The student will understand the importance of and practice asepsis, waste segregation and appropriate disposal
8. The student will understand the importance of and practice the best method to prevent the development of infection in self and patient [e.g. hand washing, using aprons for hospitals in hospitals only, regularly washing the aprons, wearing gloves while examining patients' /handling specimens, to name a few]
9. The student will understand the use of the different antimicrobial agents including antibiotics to prevent misuse [prescribing attitude]
10. The student will understand the significance of vaccinations and will receive appropriate vaccines [e.g. TT, hepatitis B and any other as per needs]
11. The student will wash his/her hands with soap and water after each practical classes.
12. The student will leave the area allotted for his practical neat and tidy.
13. The student will discard the slides in the appropriate container provided for the same.
14. The student will report any injury sustained in class, immediately.
15. The student will report any breakage occurring during class times, immediately.
16. The student may give suggestions to improve teacher-student association.

CONTENTS

Section IV: Mycology Practicals

Section V: Virology Practicals

Section VI: Parasitology Practicals

Section VII: Medical Entomology Practicals

Date:________________

PRACTICAL-1

MICROSCOPY

LEARNING OBJECTIVES:

At the end of the tutorial and practical, the student will be able to

1. List the different methods of microscopy to demonstrate microbes.
2. Explain the principles of light (compound) microscope, dark field microscope, phase contrast microscope, fluorescence microscope and electron microscope.
3. Enumerate the applications of the different microscope with specific reference to diagnostic microbiology.
4. Handle the compound light microscope appropriately.
5. List the various parts of the light microscope
6. Mention the use of the various parts and the different objectives.
7. Care for the microscope
    - Keep it dust free
    - Clean all objective lenses after use with soft cloth.
    - Oil immersion lens to be cleaned with Xylene soaked cloth.
8. Explain the following terms: definition, resolving power and magnification.
9. Define micrometry and enumerate its applications.
10. Explain the rationale behind the use of oil in oil immersion objective.

DEMONSTRATIONS:

1. Use, handling and care of microscope
2. Focusing slides under the various objectives and interpreting the same.
3. Measurement of objects (relative to size of standard cells like WBC)

PRACTICAL AND EXERCISE:

1. **Enumerate the different microscope.**

    1---2--

    3---4--

    5---6--

2. **Define Resolution power:**

----

3. **Define magnification:**

----

4. **Define Numerical aperture:**

----

5. **Define micrometry and enumerate its applications**

----

6. **Explain the principles of**

(a) Light (Compound) microscope

(b) Dark ground microscope.

(c) Fluorescence microscope.

(d) Phase contrast microscope.

(e) Electron microscope.

----

7. Give minimum two applications each of the different microscope.

   a) Light microscope:

      1. ………………………………………………………………………………

      2.………………………………………………………………………………

      ………………………………………………………………………………

b) Dark ground microscope.

1. ....

2...

....

c) Fluorescence microscope.

1. ....

2...

....

d) Phase contrast microscope.

1. ....

2...

....

e) Electron microscope.

1. ....

2...

....

8. Explain the rationale behind the use of oil in oil immersion objective

----

----

9. Draw and label the different parts of the monocular light microscope.

Date:_______________

PRACTICAL-2

MORPHOLOGY OF BACTERIA

LEARNING OBJECTIVES:

1. Mention the applications of unstained preparations.
2. Mention two important differential staining techniques.
3. Identify microscopically the different types of cells in a given stained / unstained specimen.
4. Identify correctly morphology of bacteria after staining.
5. Enumerate the methods for demonstrating the following structures of a bacterial cell viz: cell wall, spore, capsule, flagella and fimbriae.
6. Identify motile bacteria in hanging drop preparations.
7. Give two examples each of the different morphological forms of bacteria. List the methods required for studying morphology of bacteria.

DEMONSTRATIONS:

1. Smear from pus showing pus cells and Gram-positive cocci in clusters.
2. Smear of sputum from a case of pneumonia showing pus cells and Gram-positive cocci in pairs.
3. A throat swab specimen from a case of follicular tonsillitis showing Gram-positive cocci in chains along with pus cells and other bacteria.
4. Smear from a case of gonococcal pus showing Gram-negative diplococci.
5. Smear of urine showing pus cells and Gram-negative bacilli from a case of UTI.
6. Smear of pus/wound swab from a case of gas gangrene showing spore bearing/spindle shaped Gram-positive bacilli.
7. India ink preparation on capsulated pneumococci.
8. Gram-positive bacilli arranged in Chinese letter pattern suggestive of diphtheria.
9. Albert's stain of diphtheria bacilli showing metachromatic granules.
10. Fontana's film of chancroid exudate demonstrating spirochaetes.
11. Gram's stain of *Borrelia*.
12. Acid fast staining of positive sputum specimen for tubercle bacilli.
13. Hanging drop preparation to demonstrate motile bacteria.

PRACTICAL AND EXERCISE:

(Please draw your findings in the space provided and label appropriately)

1. Gram's stained smear of pus

2. Smear of sputum from a case of pneumonia

3. Smear from throat swab c/o follicular tonsillitis.

4. Smear from urethral discharge c/o gonorrhea.

5. Smear of urine from a case of UTI.

6. Smear of pus c/o gas gangrene.

7. Smear of throat swab
c/o diphtheria.

8. Albert's stain on
C. diphtheria

9. Fontana's staining of discharge
c/o chancre

10.Smear from urethral
discharge

11. Negative staining of
capsulated pneumococci.

12. Acid fast staining on tubercle bacilli.

Q. 1. Mention the applications of unstained preparations.

Q.2. Mention two important differential staining techniques.

1...

2...

Q.3. Enumerate the methods for demonstrating the following structures of a bacterial cell:

a) Cell wall..
b) Spore...
c) Capsule..
d) Flagella..
e) Fimbriae...

Q.4. Define motility and classify it:

Date:______________

PRACTICAL-3

STERILIZATION AND DISINFECTION

LEARNING OBJECTIVES:

At the end of the tutorial and practical, the student will be able to

1. Enumerate the different methods of sterilization.
2. Enumerate the different methods of sterilization by heat and know their applications.
3. Mention the temperature and time required for sterilization by heat.
4. Mention the concentration and contact time for commonly used disinfectants.
5. List 2 applications for each disinfectant with specific reference to hospitals.
6. Explain the terms sterilization, disinfection, asepsis and antisepsis.
7. Choose the most appropriate method of sterilization / disinfection for commonly used articles in the hospital and Microbiology laboratory.
8. Explain the concept of Universal safety Precautions.
9. Explain, practice and teach the concept of hygienic and surgical hand wash.
10. Enumerate the application(s) of fumigation.
11. Enumerate the uses of bacterial filters.
12. Explain the steps to render safe all articles, which will be reused in the hospital.

INTRODUCTION:

Definition of sterilization:

Sterilization is a process that destroys or eliminates all forms of microorganisms including spores on a surface, article, and culture medium or in a fluid.

Definition of disinfection:

Disinfection is a process that eliminates all pathogenic microorganisms, excluding spores.

Definition of Antiseptic:

It opposing microbial infection; especially preventing or inhibiting the growth or action of microorganisms (such as bacteria) in or on living tissue.

DEMONSTRATIONS:

1. Demonstrate the actual working of the autoclave and the use of the indicator strips / methods.
2. Familiarize the students with the working of inspissator, vaccine bath, Koch's steamer, hot air oven and biosafety cabinets.
3. Familiarize the students with the various disinfectants available in the hospital.
4. Demonstrate the in-use test for a disinfectant.

PRACTICAL AND EXERCISE:

1. Enumerate the different methods of sterilization by dry heat. Give their applications.

2. Enumerate the different methods of sterilization by moist heat. Give their applications.

3. Enumerate the different types of filtration methods. Give their applications.

4. Choose the appropriate working condition from the second column for each method in the first column.

METHOD	TEMPERATURE AND TIME	ANSWER
1. Autoclave	a. 72°C for 15 seconds followed by rapid cooling.	
2. Inspissation	b. 85°C for 30 minutes on 3 successive days.	
3. Tyndallisation	c. 160°C for 60 minutes.	
4. Koch's steamer	d. 121°C for 20 minutes.	
5. Vaccine bath	e. 100°C for 30 minutes on 3 consecutive days.	
6. Pasteurisation	f. 100°C for 30 minutes.	
7. Hot air oven	g. 60°C for 30 minutes.	

5. Choose the appropriate biological control from the second column for each method in the first column.

METHOD	BIOLOGICAL INDICATOR	ANSWER
1. Autoclave	a. *Serratia marcescens*	
2. Hot air oven	b. *Bacillus pumilus*	
3. Radiation	c. *Geobacillus stearothermophilus*	
4. Ethylene oxide	d. *Clostridium tetani*	
5. Filtration	e. *Bacillus subtilis*	

6. What are the measures to be taken before fumigating a given area in the hospital?

----

7. Enumerate Universal safety precautions.

8. Enumerate Hand washing steps given by world health organization (WHO).

9. Write the appropriate category of waste, bag/container required and treatment of that waste in respective column given to next.

Type of Waste	**Category**	**Bag/Container required**	**Treatment**
Human/animal anatomical waste, soiled waste, expired or discarded medicines, chemical solid waste, discarded linen, mattresses, beddings contaminated with blood or body fluid.			
Chemical Liquid Waste			
Microbiology laboratory waste			
Contaminated Waste (Recyclable) – plastic bag, bottles, pipes or container			
Waste sharps including Metals: needles, syringes, from needle tip cutter or burner, scalpels, blades.			
Glassware: Broken or discarded & contaminated glass – medicine vial, ampoules			
Metallic Body Implants			

10. **Guidelines for disposal of-**

a) Common antiseptics used in hospital set up (Spirit, providione-iodione, chlrhexdine)

----

b) Common disinfectants used in hospital set up (Na-hypochlorite, Lysol, Gluteraldehyde)

- Immediate measures for needle-stick/sharp injuries:
  - Don't panic.
  - Allow injured part to bleed.
  - Wash with soap and water under running tap.
  - Apply spirit / antiseptic.
  - Report immediately to concerned authority in hospital.

11. In case of hospital-acquired infections due to reuse of equipment, how would you ensure quality assurance?

----

12. Mention the working concentrations of- a) Na-hypochlorite
b) Lysol
c) Gluteraldehyde

13. How are the following articles sterilized / disinfected in the hospital?

Item	**Method of Sterilization**
Hospital linen	
Surgical gown	
Plastic syringes	
Glass syringes	
Needles	
Surgical instruments	
Endoscopes	
Culture media (solid & liquid) except LJ medium /Loeffler serum slope & sugar media	
Sugar media	
LJ medium /Loeffler serum slope	
Sera	
Cardiac catheters	
Cotton	
Oils	
Antibiotics	
Dusting powder	
Gloves	

PRINCIPLES AND METHODS OF DIAGNOSTIC MICROBIOLOGY

Date:________________

PRACTICAL-4

COLLECTION OF SPECIMENS AND PREPARATION PRIMARY AND SECONDARY SMEAR

LEARNING OBJECTIVES:

At the end of the tutorial and practical, the student will be able to

1. Specify the guidelines to diagnose infectious diseases in the laboratory.
2. Explain the guidelines of specimen collection with suitable examples.
3. Describe blood culture as a laboratory investigation.
4. Guide the patients to collect appropriate urine specimens.
5. Explain the need for specimens to be collected from different sites to diagnose systemic infections.
6. Define primary smear.
7. Mention importance of primary smear.
8. Mention 2 infections, which can be diagnosed, on primary smear examination.

INTRODUCTION:

Guidelines for specimen collection:

1. Collect material from the actual site of infection wherever possible.
2. Collect during that stage of the disease when it is likely to yield positive results.
3. Collect prior to the administration of antibiotics.
4. Collect sufficient quantity.
5. Collect aseptically in sterile screw capped / capped containers to avoid contamination and spillage.
6. Label the specimens appropriately.
7. Transport the specimen immediately to the laboratory.
8. Provide sufficient relevant clinical information to the laboratory.
9. Anaerobic collection differs from aerobic collection procedures.

Specimen transport:

To retain the viability of bacteria transport media may be essential.

Examples: Alkaline peptone water for *Vibrio cholera*
Thioglycolate broth for Anaerobes.
Stuart's transport medium for *Neisseria*.

Most specimens (except CSF) can be refrigerated up to 24 hours; if there is a likely delay in processing.

Primary smear:

Smear prepared directly from the clinical specimen can give valuable information to arrive at presumptive diagnosis of the infectious agent.

Both stained and unstained preparations can be examined.

For a smear preparation these are the following steps:

1. Label the slide: Use a wax pencil to draw a circle on the slide to help you locate the smear later.
2. Transfer a small amount of sample: Using an inoculation loop, transfer a small amount of clinical sample with wire loop to the center of the slide. If the sample is tissue/catheter tube then it can be first incubated in peptone water and then from tube, add a drop or a few loopfuls of liquid culture first and if it is swabs then directly prepare the smear with swab only.
3. Spread the sample by using the loop into a thin, even film over the circle.
4. Allow the smear to air dry completely.
5. Fix the smear: Use heat fixation to attach the smear to the slide. Heat fixation involves passing the slide through a Bunsen burner flame multiple times. Avoid prolonged heating, as it can distort the cells.

Note: A good smear preparation is essential for a good stain. Poor smear preparation is a common cause of staining errors.

DEMONSTRATIONS:

- Appropriate containers for sputum, urine, blood culture bottles, and sterile swabs.

PRACTICAL AND EXERCISE:

Answer the Following Questions.

1. What is /are the specimens to be collected from a case of pulmonary tuberculosis?

2. Describe the procedure for blood culture with specific reference to its indications, site of collection, preparation of site, mode of collection, time of collection, amount to be collected , medium and container used and processing of the specimen.

3. Describe the procedure for urine culture with specimen reference to males, females and children and the instructions to patient before collection of the sample.

4. How specimens are collected and transported for anaerobic culture?

5. How cerebral spinal fluid (CSF) specimen collected and transported for culture?

6. Define primary smear.

7. Mention importance of primary smear.

8. Mention 2 infections, which can be diagnosed, on primary smear examination.

Date:________________

PRACTICAL-5

GRAM STAINING

LEARNING OBJECTIVES:

At the end of the tutorial and practical, the student will be able to

1. Explain the limitations of microscopy to identify the infectious agent.
2. Enumerate the reagents required for Gram's staining technique.
3. Stain the given smear by Gram's staining method satisfactorily in 15 minutes within 2 attempts.
4. Interpret the staining appropriately, identifying all the cellular components and the bacteria.
5. Explain the principle of Gram's staining.

DEMONSTRATIONS:

- Reagents for Grams stain.
- Smear of pus for Gram's staining showing pus cells and Gram-positive cocci with Gram-negative bacilli.

Preparation of smears:

The material to study is spread evenly on a clean, grease free glass slide by using sterile inoculation loop or sterile swab. The smear is then air dried or fixed by gentle heating.

9. Describe the method of Gram's staining.

a) Principle of Gram stain:

b) Procedure of Gram stain:

10. Draw and label the findings of the smear that you have stained.

c) Interpretation:

d) Explain Modified Gram stain

11. Give 5 examples of each (aerobic and anaerobic):

- Gram-positive cocci:

  1...

  2...

  3...

  4...

  5...

- Gram-positive bacilli:

  1...

  2...

  3...

  4...

  5...

- Gram-negative cocci:

  1...

  2...

  3...

  4...

  5...

- Gram-negative bacilli:

  1...

  2...

  3...

  4...

  5...

Date:__________________

PRACTICAL-6

ACID FAST (ZN) STAINING

LEARNING OBJECTIVES:

At the end of the tutorial and practical, the student will be able to

1. Explain the limitations of microscopy to identify the infectious agent.
2. Enumerate the reagents required for modified acid-fast staining technique.
3. Stain the given smear by modified acid-fast staining method satisfactorily in 30 minutes within 2 attempts.
4. Interpret the staining appropriately, identifying all the cellular components and the bacteria.
5. Explain the principle of acid fast staining.

Primary smear:

Smear prepared directly from the clinical specimen can give valuable information to arrive at presumptive diagnosis of the infectious agent.

Both stained and unstained preparations can be examined.

DEMONSTRATIONS:

- Reagents for Acid fast stain.
- Smear of sputum showing 1+, 2+ and 3+ acid-fast bacilli.

PRACTICAL

1. Describe the method of acid fast staining.

   a) Principle of ZN stain

   b) Procedure of ZN stain

2. Draw and label the findings of the smear that you have stained.

c) Interpretation of ZN stain:

d) Modification in ZN stain:

3. Give 7 examples of acid fast microorganisms

1……………………………………………………………………………………

2……………………………………………………………………………………

3……………………………………………………………………………………

4……………………………………………………………………………………

5……………………………………………………………………………………

6……………………………………………………………………………………

7……………………………………………………………………………………

4. Microscopic Grading for Mycobacterium tuberculosis (in pulmonary tuberculosis) Please write appropriate grading of each number of bacilli also mention how many fields required to be examined for different grades.

Number of bacilli	Grade	Number of fields to be examined
No AFB in 100 oil immersion fields		
1-9 AFB per 100 oil immersion fields		
10-99 AFB per 100 oil immersion fields		
1-10 AFB per oil immersion field		
More than 10 AFB per oil immersion field		

5. Please describe the importance of grading of Mycobacterium tuberculosis in case of pulmonary TB.

___

___

___

___

___

6. What is DOTS, RNTCP, NTEP (write the full form)

DOTS……………………………………………………………………………………

RNTCP……………………………………………………………………………………

NTEP……………………………………………………………………………………

Date:________________

PRACTICAL-7

ALBERT STAINING

LEARNING OBJECTIVES:

At the end of the tutorial and practical, the student will be able to

1. Enumerate the reagents required for Albert staining technique.
2. Stain the given smear by Albert staining method satisfactorily in 15 minutes within 2 attempts.
3. Interpret the staining appropriately, identifying all the cellular components and the bacteria.
4. Explain the principle of Albert stain.

Primary smear:

Smear prepared directly from the clinical specimen can give valuable information to arrive at presumptive diagnosis of the infectious agent.

DEMONSTRATIONS:

- Reagents for Albert stain.
- Smear of throat swab showing Chinese letter patter arrangement.

PRACTICAL:

1. Describe the method of acid fast staining.

   a) Principle of Albert stain

b) Procedure of Albert stain

2. Draw and label the findings of the smear that you have stained.

c) Interpretation of Albert stain:

Date:_________________

PRACTICAL-8

OTHER STAINING

LEARNING OBJECTIVES:

At the end of the tutorial and practical, the student will be able to

1. Specify the staining techniques for capsule, spores, and flagella.
2. Specify the staining technique used for Treponema.

INTRODUCTION

Treponema is typically stained using silver impregnation techniques, such as Warthin-Starry, Levaditi, or Dieterle modified by Steiner. However, Treponema bacteria are Gram-negative, but they don't stain easily with Gram or Giemsa staining.

Dark-field microscopy: Used to visualize live treponemes.

DEMONSTRATIONS:

- Reagents for negative staining, sliver impregnation staining.
- Smear of pus for Silver impregnation stain showing pus cells and spiral coiled bacteria.

PRACTICAL

1. Draw and label the findings of the negative staining demonstrated to you

2. Draw and label the findings of the silver impregnation staining demonstrated to you

3. Enumerate the different types of staining techniques that can be done to visualize bacteria.

EXTRA SPACE

PRINCIPLES AND METHODS OF DIAGNOSTIC MICROBIOLOGY

Date:__________________

PRACTICAL-9

ISOLATION OF ORGANISMS, THEIR IDENTIFICATION AND ANTIBIOTIC SUSCEPTIBILITY TESTING.

LEARNING OBJECTIVES:

At the end of the tutorial and practical, the student will be able to

1. Enumerate the methods used for the isolation of organisms in pure culture.
2. List the application of isolation.
3. Define a nutrient medium.
4. List the growth requirements of bacteria.
5. Classify bacteria based on their growth requirements.
6. Classify media and explain the terms enriched, enrichment, defined, selective, differential, simple, complex giving suitable examples and their applications.
7. Identify Blood agar, MacConkey's agar, Chocolate agar, and Nutrient agar.
8. Recognize and describe the colony characteristics on blood agar, nutrient agar and MacConkey's agar, Staphylococci, Streptococci (haemolytic/ non-haemolytic, pigmented, LF and NLF).
9. Mention the methods of sterilization of commonly used media.
10. Enumerate the commonly used biochemical tests for identification of bacteria.
11. Explain the reason for the use of biochemical tests for identification.
12. Applications and limitations of laboratory animals (Rabbit, Guinea Pig, Rat and Mouse) in diagnostic microbiology
13. Explain the reasons for the performance of antimicrobial susceptibility testing on all clinical isolates.
14. Enumerate the different methods of antimicrobial susceptibility testing giving suitable examples.
15. Define MIC and MBC.
16. Enumerate the limitations of in vitro susceptibility tests.
17. Interpret Kirby Bauer disk diffusion tests.

INTRODUCTION:

Organisms are isolated in the laboratory directly from the clinical specimens. The specimens are inoculated onto appropriate media by making use of sterile Nichrome wire loops under aseptic conditions. These plates are incubated appropriately depending upon the gaseous requirement of the organism under consideration (aerobic / anaerobic / capnophilic) and optimum temperature.

To diagnose infective diseases it is necessary to collect appropriate specimen(s) from the actual site of infection.

1. Perform a primary smear examination.
2. Cultivate the organism on appropriate media since this has greater sensitivity.
3. Identify the organism isolated from the specimen.
4. Perform antimicrobial susceptibility test on the isolate.

Bacteria are identified based on their cultural characteristics. Some bacteria however share similar cultural characteristics and hence can be identified only by their specific biochemical properties. For example: *Streptococcus pneumoniae*, a potential respiratory pathogen produces alpha haemolytic colonies on blood agar, a property shared by the normal commensals of the oropharynx, *Streptococcus viridians*.

The biochemical tests are based on the capacity of the organisms to break down sugars and proteins and / or the presence of specific enzymes like catalase, oxidase etc.

DEMONSTRATIONS:

1. Laboratory animals: white rat, white mouse, guinea pig and rabbit.
2. Uninoculated: Blood agar, MacConkey's agar, Nutrient agar, and Chocolate agar.
   F broth, Alkaline peptone water
   Robertson's cooked meat medium, Thioglycolate broth.
3. Inoculated: Blood agar, MacConkey's agar and Disc diffusion on Muller Hinton Agar.
   Pigmented colonies of *Staphylococcus* species on Nutrient agar.
4. Demonstration of oxidase test, TSI uninoculated and showing acid, gas and H_2S production.

PRACTICAL AND EXERCISE:

Q.1 Enumerate two advantages each of liquid medium and solid medium.

a) Liquid Medium:

1____

2____

b) Solid Medium

1____

2____

Q.2 Give five examples of liquid medium.

1____

2____

3____

4____

5____

Q.3 Give two examples of each of the following:

a) Enriched medium– ______________________________

b) Enrichment medium– ______________________________

c) Selective medium– ______________________________

d) Differential medium– ______________________________

e) Simple medium– ______________________________

f) Defined medium– ______________________________

g) Transport medium– ______________________________

Q.4 Enumerate two commonly used ingredients for solidifying liquid media.

Q.5 How blood agar is prepared?

Q.6 Enumerate the essential components of MacConkey's agar.

Q.7 Draw the following media.

1) Blood agar with α haemolysis.
2) Blood agar with β haemolysis.
3) MacConkey's agar with lactose fermenting colonies.
4) Chocolate agar.
5) Nutrient agar.
6) Lowenstein-Jensen medium.

1. Blood agar with α haemolysis.

2. Blood agar with β haemolysis.

3. MacConkey's agar with lactose fermenting colonies.

4. Chocolate agar

5. Nutrient agar

6. L-J Medium

Q.8 Draw the various reactions on Triple Sugar Iron Agar demonstrated to you.

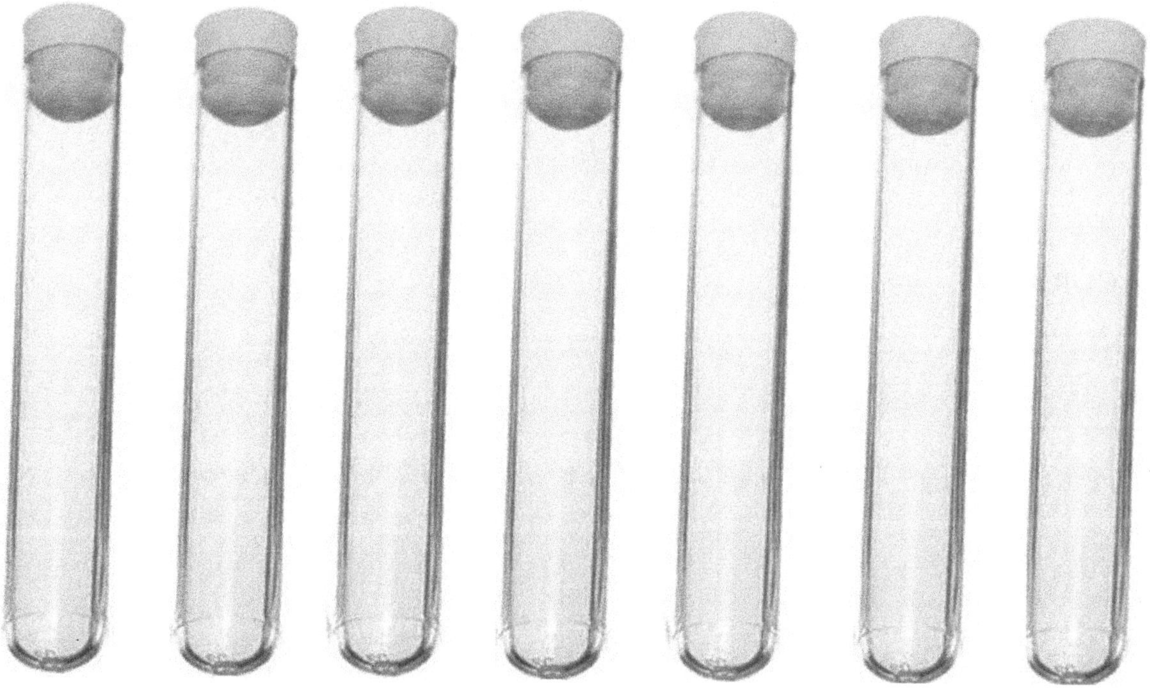

Un-inoculated A/A A/A with gas A/A with H_2S K/A K/A with gas K/A with H_2S

Q.9 Enumerate the laboratory uses of the following animals.

A) White mouse

B) Guinea pig

C) Rabbit

Q.10 Describe Kirby-Bauer disc diffusion methods of antimicrobial susceptibility testing.

Q.11 Describe breakpoint in antibiotic susceptibility testing (AST).

Q.12 Enumerate the factors affecting in-vitro susceptibility tests.

Q.13 Enumerate four bactericidal and four bacteriostatic agents.

Bactericidal agents

1 ______________________________

2 ______________________________

3 ______________________________

4 ______________________________

Bacteriostatic agents

1 ______________________________

2 ______________________________

3 ______________________________

4 ______________________________

Q.14 Draw and label the disk diffusion test demonstrated to you and interpret the same.

IMMUNOLOGY

Date:_______________

PRACTICAL-10

IMMUNOLOGICAL AND SEROLOGICAL METHODS FOR THE DIAGNOSIS OF INFECTIOUS DISEASES

LEARNING OBJECTIVES:

At the end of the tutorial and practical, the student will be able to

1. Explain the role of serology in the diagnosis of infectious diseases.
2. Enumerate the advantages and disadvantages of serological diagnosis.
3. Enumerate the different types of serological tests.
4. Explain the principles of the different serological tests.
5. Enumerate the applications of the various serological tests.
6. Explain the terms-specificity, sensitivity, titre and biological false positive reactions.
7. Enumerate the different methods for detecting CMI.

INTRODUCTION:

Infectious diseases can be diagnosed by

1. Documenting the presence of the infective agent in the patient, by microscopy and / or culture / or nucleic detection methods like PCR.
2. By detecting a specific product of the infectious agent in the patient.
3. By detecting a specific immunological response.

We have seen the applications of the first two in the previous practicals.

Immunological response is of two types:

- Cell mediated and
- Antibody mediated.

The patient's serum is tested for specific antibody response. Serum can also be used for detecting antigens in specific infections: HBsAg, MTB etc. Material from the site of infection /where the organism may be present is used for detecting antigens.

Serological reactions are antigen antibody reactions between corresponding antigens and antibodies, taking place in vitro at an optimum pH, temperature and in the presence of electrolytes.

The reactions between antigen and antibody occur in 3 stages.

I. The primary stage, where there is no visible reaction. Can be detected by measuring free antigen or antibody by ELISA, RIA or Immunoflourescence.

II. The secondary stage where visible reactions occur viz: precipitation, agglutination, neutralization, complement fixation and opsonisation.

III. The tertiary stage, in certain infections is characterized by persistent antigenemia.

DEMONSTRATIONS:

1. Precipitation in gel (slide)
    - Counter-current immunoelectrophoresis
    - VDRL/TRUST/RPR

2. Agglutination:
    - Llatex (RA) agglutination,
    - Hhaemagglutination,
    - Indirect Haemagglutination
    - Widal test

3. ELISA
4. Neutralization: ASO test
5. Tuberculin test.

PRACTICAL AND EXERCISE:

Q.1. Enumerate the different serological tests.

Q.2. Explain the terms specificity, sensitivity and titre.

Specificity

Sensitivity

Titre

Q.3. Explain the principles of the following serological reactions and enumerate applications of each.

Precipitation: (Counter-current immunoelectrophoresis, VDRL/TRUST/RPR)

a) Agglutination (Latex agglutination (RA), Haemagglutination, IHA, Widal):

Complement fixation:

b) Neutralization:

c) Radioimmunoassay (RIA)

d) ELISA: Principle, Procedure, Type and Applications

e) Fluorescent antibody tests.

Q.4. Enumerate the different types of precipitation reactions giving applications of each

Q.5. Enumerate the different types of agglutination reaction, giving applications of each

Q.6. How and why is serum inactivated?

Q.7. What is the importance of antigen detection test?

Q.8. What is the significance of quantitation in serology?

Q.9. Enumerate the serological test to diagnose neonatal infection?

Q.10. Explain the term biological false positive reaction giving suitable examples.

Q.11 What is prozone phenomenon?

Q.12 What is post zone phenomenon?

Q.13 Enumerate the methods for detecting CMI

EXTRA SPACE

SYSTEMIC BACTERIOLOGY

LEARNING OBJECTIVES :

At the end of the tutorial and practical, the student will be able to:

1. Enumerate the infections produced by the organism.
2. Enumerate the different virulence factors, explaining their mode of action
3. Enumerate the important clinical features of the various infections.
4. Explain the pathogenesis of infections due to a given organism.
5. Describe the morphology of the organism.
6. List the important media used and the mode for cultivating them.
7. Explain the different steps involved in the laboratory diagnosis of infections caused by the organism.
8. Enumerate the drugs of choice for therapy and the method for testing the same.
9. Explain the importance of antimicrobial susceptibility testing.
10. Identify the organism in primary smears based on their Gram's staining properties.
11. Interpret the given antibiotic susceptibility test.
12. Identify the selective media and describe the colony characteristics of the organism on specific media where applicable.

Date:________________

PRACTICAL-11

STAPHYLOCOCCI

LEARNING OBJECTIVES:

At the end of the tutorial and practical, the student will be able to

1. Classify Staphylococci based on virulence and pigment production
2. List the differences between pathogenic and non-pathogenic Staphylococci.
3. Describe the role of Staphylococci in nosocomial infections and the importance of typing.
4. Differentiate the different pigment producing strains on culture media.
5. What is MRSA and its significance?

INTRODUCTION:

These are aerobic or facultative anaerobic Gram-positive cocci arranged in clusters. *Staphylococcus aureus* and *Staphylococcus epidermidis* are the two important species.

PATHOGENESIS:

Host:

- The infection is normally prevented by normal flora of skin and mucosa, antibacterial substances present in blood and an intact skin.
- Staphylococci form normal commensals of the anterior nares, perineum and other skin sites in 10 - 15% of normal healthy individuals.
- Infection is transmitted via fomites and food contaminated with Staphylococcal toxin.

Agent: Staphylococcal are capable of causing pyaemic infections at various sites.

Infection caused:

- Pyaemic infections of skin and deep sites (respiratory, intestinal, cardiac, bone and joint, CNS and blood stream).
- Toxin mediated food poisoning, skin exfoliation and toxic shock syndrome
- Hospital acquired infections.

DEMONSTRATIONS:

1. A primary smear from a case of abscess stained by Gram's stain showing pus cells and Gram-positive cocci in clusters.
2. Growth characteristics of the different pigment producers on Nutrient agar.
3. Growth characteristics of haemolytic and non-haemolytic Staphylococci.
4. Antibiotic sensitivity test showing sensitive and resistant strains by the Kirby Bauer method.
5. Coagulase positive and negative test.
6. Detection of beta lactamase production.

PRACTICAL AND EXERCISE:

1. Do Gram's stain on the smear from a specimen of pus and report your findings.

2. Draw antibiotic sensitivity testing of *Staphylococcus aureus* and interpret it.

3. Draw the different pigment producing stains of Staphylococci.

4. A 45-year-old known non-insulin dependent diabetic patient presents with history of recurrent pyaemic lesions.

   a) What is the probable infective agent?

   b) How will you arrive at the diagnosis?

   c) What is the significance of hospital-associated infections?

Date:________________

PRACTICAL- 12

STREPTOCOCCI

LEARNING OBJECTIVES:

At the end of the tutorial and practical, the student will be able to:

1. Classify Streptococci.
2. Enumerate the non-suppurative complications following infection due to Streptococcus pyogenes and explain their pathogenesis.
3. Enumerate the important antigens of Streptococci.
4. List the infections produced by the different Groups of Streptococci.
5. Identify and describe the colony characteristics of Streptococci.
6. List the methods used for demonstrating the capsulated Strep-pneumoniae.
7. Enumerate the organisms producing alpha haemolysis on blood agar.
8. List the differences between Streptococcus pneumoniae and Streptococcus viridians.
9. Explain the role of Streptococcus viridians in health and disease.
10. Interpret the given antibiotic susceptibility test.
11. Identify the ASO test.
12. Mention the principle, application and the diagnostic titre of the ASO test.

INTRODUCTION:

This genus consists of Gram-positive cocci arranged in chains, which are aerobic or facultative anaerobic. They cause both suppurative infections, as well as non-suppurative complications. They include the beta haemolytic Streptococcus pyogenes, the alpha hemolytic Streptococcus pneumoniae and the non-haemolytic variants.

PATHOGENESIS:

Host:

It forms the normal nasopharyngeal and oropharyngeal flora in 10-15% of children and 5% of adults.

Predisposing factors include viral infections of Respiratory Tract, Silicosis and alcoholism.

Agent:

The virulence factors for Streptococcus pneumoniae include

The capsular polysaccharide-antiphagocytic

Pneumolysins – cytoloytic

Neuraminidase –degrades surface structure of host tissue and

C substance –which activates non-specific defense mechanisms

The virulence factors of Strep-pyogenes are:

M.protein	-	antiphagocytic
Hyaluronidase	-	spread of infection
DNAse	-	cell death
Streptokinase	-	breaks down clots
Streptolysin O and S	-	cytolytic
Cell wall lipoteichoic acid	-	adherence to host cell respiratory epithelium.

Infections produced:

- Suppurative: Acute infections of the respiratory tract, skin, gynaecological, sepsis and lymphadenitis.
- The non-suppurative complications include: Rheumatic fever, Rheumatic heart disease and acute glomerulonephritis.

DEMONSTRATIONS:

1. A Gram's stained smear of a case of follicular tonsillitis showing predominant Gram-positive cocci in chains along with cellular elements and microbial flora.
2. Cultural characteristics of Strep. Pyogenes and Strep. Pneumoniae on blood agar.
3. A Gram's stained smear of C.S.F from a case of pneumococcal meningitis.
4. Antibiotic susceptibility pattern of Streptococcus pyogenes, which is sensitive to Penicillins, and Streptococcus pneumonia, which may show resistance.
5. India ink preparation showing capsulated pneumococci.
6. A diagnostic ASO test.

PRACTICAL AND EXERCISE:

1. Gram's stain of throat swab form a c/o follicular tonsillitis

2. Gram's stain of CSF from a c/o pneumococcal meningitis

3. Blood agar showing alpha hemolytic colonies of Streptococcus viridians

4. Blood agar showing beta hemolytic colonies of Streptococcus pyogenes

3. Report the findings of the antimicrobial susceptibility test of Streptococcus pyogenes and Streptococcus pneumoniae demonstrated to you.

4. Draw a sensitive and resistant on Optochin (ethylhydrocupreine hydrochloride) and bacitracin on disc also mention the species name.

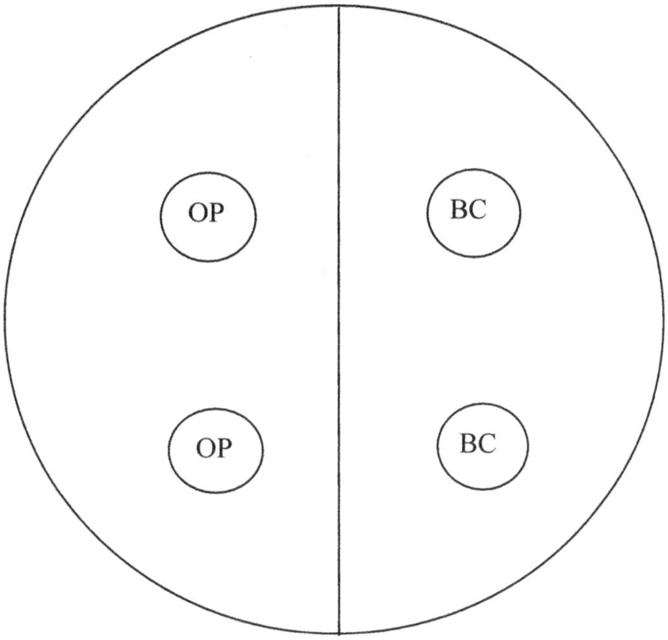

5. Draw a diagram of Christie-Atkinson-Munch-Peterson (CAMP) test and describe the test in brief.

6. A 7-year-old male child presents with past history of recurrent episodes of upper respiratory tract infections and presently complains of knee joint pain and swelling. How will you arrive at the diagnosis of rheumatic fever?

7. Enumerate 4 bacteria causing upper & lower respiratory tract infection.

Date:________________

PRACTICAL -13
NEISSERIAE

LEARNING OBJECTIVES:

At the end of the tutorial and practical, the student will be able to:

1. Classify Neisseria.
2. Enumerate the complications following infection due to Neisseria gonorrhoeae.
3. List the differences between *N. meningitidis* and *N. gonorrhoeae.*
4. Explain the different steps involved in the laboratory diagnosis of meningitis and gonorrhoeae.
5. Enumerate the rapid test that will aid diagnosis.

INTRODUCTION:

The Neisseriae are aerobic Gram-negative cocci, which appear in stained preparations as diplococci.

The genus contains two potential pathogens, Neisseria gonorrhoeae which causes gonorrhoeae, a sexually transmitted disease and *N. meningitides,* which causes meningitis, a potentially fatal infection if not promptly treated.

Pathogenesis

1. GONORRHOEA

Host: Man is the only natural host for *N. gonorrhoeae.*

Neonates become infected while passing through the birth canal of an infected mother.

The normal flora of the genitourinary tract prevents colonisation by this organism.

Carrier states in both men and women occur.

Agent: the organisms adhere by means of pili and also elaborate IgA proteases which decrease the local immunity.

Infections: Gonorrhoea, ophthalmia neonatorum and disseminated disease.

2. MENINGITIS:

N. meningitidis attach by means of adherence factors to nasopharyngeal and oropharyngeal mucosa and locally multiply.

They then invade the blood stream and enter CSF producing meningitis in non-immune individuals.

DEMONSTRATIONS:

1. A Gram's stained smear of the urethral exudate from a case of gonorrhoea.
2. A Gram's stained smear of C.S.F from a case of meningitis
3. Growth on chocolate agar of *N. gonorrhoeae* and *N. meningitidis* showing characteristic colonies.
4. Key biochemical reaction (oxidase)
5. Antimicrobial susceptibility pattern of the strains on the chocolate agar medium.

PRATICAL AND EXERCISE:

Gram's stained smear of Urethral Pus

Gram's stained smear of CSF

1. What is Waterhouse-Friderichson syndrome?

2. A 13-year-old patient arrives with c/o acute onset fever, toxaemia and vomiting and confusion. On examination, neck rigidity and Kernig's sign are positive. There are purpuric spots on the skin.

a) What is / are the causative agent/s?

b) How will you arrive at the diagnosis?

3. Write down your findings of the Antimicrobial susceptibility pattern of *N. gonorrhoeae* and *N. meningitidis*.

Date:________________

PRACTICAL-14

CORYNEBACTERIA

LEARNING OBJECTIVES:

At the end of the tutorial and practical, the student will be able to

1. Explain the principle of the Schick test.
2. List the other non-diphtheria Corynebateria and mention their associated infections.
3. List the important vaccines.
4. Explain the role of laboratory animals with specific reference to diphtheria.

INTRODUCTION:

Corynebateria are non-spore forming Gram-positive rods. Corynebacterium diphtheria is the most important species in this genus. C. diphtheriae causes a very well-known pediatric disease called 'Diphtheria'.

C. diphtheriae causes sore throat and the bacteria are confined to throat. They produce a necrotic toxin, which leads to causes necrosis of mucosa at the site of infection. Inflammatory exudate, tissue debries, pus cell etc. are entangled in the fibrinous net work at the site locally where C. diphtheriae continue to multiply and a thick leathery membrane is formed. The toxin is also absorbed in blood and toxemia is produced. Diphtheria is basically toxemia. The toxin has specific action on heart muscle, nerve endings and the adrenal glands. The toxin acts by inhibition of protein synthesis. Without early clinical diagnosis and prompt treatment the disease may be fatal.

The organism C. diphtheriae is originally not toxigenic but when it is infected with beta phage it is lysogenically converted to the toxigenic variety. In laryngeal diphtheriae the tough leathery membrane can cause severe respiratory obstruction and may lead to death.

DEMONSTRATIONS:

1. Gram stained smear of C. diphtheriae.

2. Albert stained smear of C. diphtheriae
3. Growth of C.d. on Loffler's serum slope.
4. Growth of C.d. on Potassium telluride medium.
5. Vial of DPT vaccine.
6. Vial of DT vaccine.
7. Vial of ADS.
8. Guinea pig.
9. Rabbit.

PRACTICAL AND EXERCISE:

Q1. Which specimen is collected for the laboratory diagnosis of diphtheria?

Q2. Draw a diagram of Gram stained and Albert stained smear of *C. diphtheriae*.

Q. 3 Describe the morphology of *C. diphtheriae*.

Q. 4 Mention the importance of Loeffler's serum slope and Potassium tellurite agar in the laboratory diagnosis of diphtheria

Q.5 Mention the three main biotypes of C. diphtheriae and give importance of each of them in one sentence each

Q6. How do you toxigenicity of C. diphtheriae?

Q7. Draw a diagram of Elek's test and describe the test in brief.

Q.8 Mention the immunization against diphtheria.

Date:________________

PRACTICAL- 15

BACILLUS

LEARNING OBJECTIVES:

At the end of the tutorial and practical, the student will be able to

1. Enumerate the important member of this genus associated with human infections.
2. Enumerate the important infections produced by anthrax in man.
3. Will explain the principle and application of Ascoli's test.
4. Will explain the laboratory diagnosis of B. cereus food poisoning.

INTRODUCTION:

The genus *Bacillus* includes large Gram-positive, spore forming, aerobic rods. They form heat resistant spores. *Bacillus* are mainly saprophytic and some species are useful as sources of antibiotics. They are frequently encountered contaminants of culture media in the laboratory. A few species are medically important e.g. *Bacillus anthracis*, the causative agent of an important zoonotic disease 'Anthrax', and *B. cereus* - causative agent of food poisoning .Some of the other important species are:

- *B. stearothermophilus*- biological indicator for testing autoclaving
- *B. subtilis*- test organism for Ethylene Oxide sterilization
- *B. pumilus*- to test efficiency of ionizing radiation methods of sterilization
- *B. polymyxa*- source of antibiotic Polymyxin.

DEMONSTRATIONS:

- Smear of *B. anthracis*
- Smear of *B. subtilis*
- Smear showing McFadyean's reaction

PRACTICAL AND EXERCISE:

Q.1. What is "Anthrax'?

Q.2. Enumerate the various lesions produced by B. anthracis in human beings.

Q3. Mention in brief the laboratory diagnosis of human Anthrax.

Q.4. Draw and label a diagram of B. anthracis seen on Gram stain and McFadyean's reaction and describe in brief.

Q.5. Draw a medusa head colonies of Bacillus anthracis on nutrient agar?

Q.6. What is Ascoli's thermoprecipitation test?

Q.7. Mention in brief prophylaxis of Anthrax.

Date:________________

PRACTICAL-16

MYCOBACTERIUM TUBERCULOSIS & NON-TUBERCULOUS MYCOBACTERIA

LEARNING OBJECTIVES:

At the end of the tutorial and practical, the student will be able to:

1. Explain the principle, application, interpretation and limitation of Mantoux test.
2. Explain the role of laboratory animals with specific reference to tuberculosis.
3. Enumerate the tests, which will differentiate MTB complex from atypical Mycobacteria.
4. List the recent advances in the laboratory diagnosis of tuberculosis.
5. Perform the acid-fast stain of the given smear in not more than 2 attempts and within 20 minutes and interpret the findings.
6. Explain the importance of microscopy in the laboratory diagnosis of tuberculosis.
7. Explain the advantages and limitations of culture.
8. Explain the relevance of multiple specimens to facilitate diagnosis.

INTRODUCTION:

Mycobacteria are the bacteria having distinctive biological characters differentiating them from most other microorganisms. Because of waxy cell wall, the Mycobacteria are not easily stained but treatment with hot carbol fuchsin stains the bacilli so fast that acid or alcohol does not decolorize them. Degree of acid fastness varies with different members of the species.

Common acid-fast bacilli (AFB)

I. Pathogenic

A. *Mycobacterium tuberculosis*
   1) Human type
   2) Bovine type
   3) Avian type
   4) Murine type
   5) Cold blooded type

B. Atypical Mycobacteria / Non-tuberculous Mycobacteria

C. *Mycobacterium leprae*

II. Non-pathogenic

1) *Mycobacterium smegmatis*
2) *Mycobacterium butyricum*
3) *Mycobacterium phlei*
4) *Mycobacterium stercoris*

DEMONSTRATIONS:

1. Acid fast stained smear of sputum showing acid-fast bacilli.
2. Culture on LJ medium of *M. tuberculosis* and pigmented atypical Mycobacteria.
3. A dissected guinea pig showing characteristic tuberculous lesions after experimental infection with tubercle bacilli.
4. Purified protein derivative and tuberculin syringe.
5. Smear made from a specimen of sputum for acid-fast stain.
6. BCG vaccine.
7. Niacin and Nitrate reduction test.

PRACTICAL AND EXERCISE:

Q1. Mention the important lesions produced by *M. tuberculosis*.

____
____
____
____
____
____
____

Q2. Mention four important clinical signs and symptoms of pulmonary tuberculosis.

____
____
____
____

Q3. Which samples will you collect for the laboratory diagnosis of pulmonary tuberculosis? How and when is it collected?

Q4. Draw a labeled diagram of sputum smear showing AFB.

Q.5. Describe briefly the morphology of *M. tuberculosis*.

Q.6. Which is a most commonly used alternative staining method for *M. tuberculosis*?

Q.7. How is *M. tuberculosis* cultured? Mention the culture medium, its important ingredients and sterilization.

Q.8. Mention the important biochemical tests for the identification of *M. tuberculosis*?

Q.9. What is radiometric culture?

Q.10. Which animals are useful in the laboratory diagnosis of tuberculosis?

Q.11. What is tuberculin test? What are its uses?

Q.12. Describe BCG vaccine.

Q.13. What is the clinical importance of atypical mycobacteria?

Q.14. Classify the atypical mycobacteria / non-tuberculous mycobacteria with examples.

Date:________________

PRACTICAL-17

MYCOBACTERIUM LEPRAE

LEARNING OBJECTIVES:

At the end of the tutorial and practical, the student will be able to

1. Explain the principle, application, interpretation and limitation of Lepromin test.
2. Enumerate the differences between tuberculoid and lepromatous leprosy.
3. Explain the role of laboratory animals in relation to leprosy.
4. Explain the terms morphological and bacteriological index and know their relevance.
5. Mention the staining technique used to demonstrate the lepra bacilli.

INTRODUCTION:

M. leprae, the causative agent of leprosy is an obligate human pathogen. It tends to display intracellular existence more frequently than *M. tuberculosis*. It is less acid fast. Leprosy is a chronic disease and it affects mainly the skin and peripheral nerves. The clinical presentation of the disease varies from person to person depending upon the degree of cell mediate immunity possessed by the patient.

DEMONSTRATIONS:

1. An acid fast stained smear of skin showing lepra bacilli.

PRACTICAL AND EXERCISE:

Q.1. Mention the specimens collected from a patient for laboratory diagnosis of leprosy.

a) --

b) --

c) --

d) --

e) --

f) --

Q.2. Draw and label a diagram of the smear of *M. leprae* demonstrated to you. Mention the percentage of Sulphuric Acid used for decolourisation in ZN staining of *M. leprae*.

Q3. Enumerate two important animals used to culture *M. leprae* also mention the route of inoculation.

Q.4. What is bacteriological index? Give an example how to calculate it.

Q.5. What is morphological index? Give an example how to calculate it.

____

____

____

____

____

____

Q.6. Microscopic grading for Mycobacterium leprae. Please write appropriate grading of each number of bacilli.

Number of bacilli	Grade
1-10 bacilli per 100 oil immersion fields	
1-10 bacilli per 10 oil immersion fields	
1-10 bacilli per oil immersion fields	
10-100 bacilli per oil immersion field	
100-1000 bacilli per oil immersion field	
>1000 bacilli, clumps & globi per oil immersion field	

Q.7. Please describes the importance of grading of Mycobacterium leprae.

____

____

____

____

____

Q.8. What is Lepromin test? What are its uses?

____

____

____

____

____

____

____

Date:________________

PRACTICAL-18

ESCHERICHIA COLI, KLEBSIELLA AND PROTEUS

LEARNING OBJECTIVES:

At the end of the tutorial and practical, the student will be able to

1. Explain the laboratory diagnosis of a case of urinary tract infection.
2. Enumerate the different types of *E. coli* and mention their pathogenesis.
3. Explain the role of these organisms in hospital acquired infections.

INTRODUCTION:

The family Enterobacteriaceae includes Gram-negative bacteria colonizing the human intestine. They are universally distributed. We are concerned in medical bacteriology with those Gram-negative bacilli, which are commonly found in the human intestine, often as commensals, and those intestinal pathogens, which are present in certain pathological conditions and occasionally in faces of healthy persons and animal reservoirs. The important genera of Enterobacteriaceae are:

1. Genus *Escherichia*: e.g. *E. coli.* This constitutes the normal bacterial flora of the intestine but some types are responsible for infantile diarrhea and urinary tract infections. They are also involved in wound infections.
2. Genus salmonella; e.g. *S. typhi, S paratyphi* A, B, C, responsible for typhoid and paratyphoid fever. *S tyhimurium* and *S. enteritidis*- responsible for acute gastroenteritis (food poisoning)
3. Genus Shigella: e.g. *S. dysenteriae*, *S. sonnei*, *S. boydii* and *S. flexneri* responsible for bacillary dysentery.
4. Genus *Klebsiella*: e.g. *K. pneumoniae, K. aerogenes* responsible for pneumonia, UTI and opportunistic pyogenic infections and wound infections.
5. Genus *Proteus*: e.g. *Proteus mirabilis, P. vulgaris* responsible for UTI and opportunistic pyogenic infections and would infection

To confirm the clinical diagnosis and to know the specific bacterial agents responsible for the above named diseases, it is essential to know the bacteriology of the disease, the source, the mode of infection and distribution of the organisms in the body.

DEMONSTRATIONS:

1. Gram's stained smear of *E. coli, Klebsiella* and *Proteus*.
2. Motility of Proteus and non-motility of *Klebsiella*.
3. Growth characteristics on blood agar and MacConkey's agar.
4. Antibiotic susceptibility pattern of the isolates.
5. Biochemical tests that help in differentiating the 3 genera. (IMViC)

PRACTICAL AND EXERCISE:

1. Draw the Gram's stained smear of *Escherichia*, *Klebsiella* & *Proteus* demonstrated.

2. Draw the colony characteristics of *E. coli* on MacConkey's agar. Describe colonies of Klebssiella and E. coli in brief.

3. Draw the colony characteristics of *Proteus* species on blood agar.

4. A 25 year old female patient comes with complains of frequency of urination, dysuria and fever with chills since 3 days. How will you arrive at the infective aetiology.

5. Mention 5 main types of diarrheagenic E. coli. Describe in brief what they cause.

6. What is swarming growth of Proteus. How to inhibit it on culture plate? Give the examples of all bacteria exhibiting swarming growth on culture plate.

7. Enumerate 4 antibiotics used for the treatment of UTI.

i. --

ii. --

iii. --

iv. --

8. Enumerate 4 bacteria causing urinary tract infection.

i. --

ii. --

iii. --

iv. --

Date:_______________

PRACTICAL - 19

SALMONELLA

LEARNING OBJECTIVES:

At the end of the tutorial and practical, the student will be able to

1. List the specimens to be collected from a case of typhoid fever, septicaemia and food poisoning.
2. Explain the relevance of the different specimens.
3. Explain the application and processing of blood culture.
4. Explain the principle, application, interpretation and limitations of the Widal test.

INTRODUCTION:

- Salmonella are Gram-negative aerobic, motile rods that are infective to humans or animals by the oral route.
- Enteric fever: includes fever caused by *Salmonella typhi*, *paratyphi* A, B, C.
- Source of infection is usually contaminated food and drink, milk and milk products,
- Shell fish from contaminated water dried or frozen eggs of infected fowls (cause Salmonellosis),
- Meat and meat product of infected animals all of which occurs as a zoonoses.
- Water contaminated with faeces can lead to explosive epidemics.
- After ingestion, there occurs primary and secondary bacteraemia and multiplication of the organism in bile and Payer's patches. The organisms multiply in the cells of the reticuloendothelial system and can only be eliminated with effective cell mediated immunity.

DEMONSTRATIONS:

1. Gram's stained smear of *Salmonella*.
2. Hanging drop preparation to demonstrate their motility.
3. Blood culture bottle.

4. Widal test.
5. Biochemical tests for species differentiation.
6. MacConkey's agar plate showing non-lactose fermenting colonies of *Salmonella*.
7. Wilson and Blair bismuth sulphite agar showing blackening of the colonies due to growth of *Salmonella typhi* and *paratyphi* B and green colonies of *paratyphi* A.
8. Selenite F and tetrathionate broth.
9. Antimicrobial susceptibility test showing sensitive strain and multidrug resistant strain.

PRACTICAL AND EXERCISE:

1. Draw the colony characteristic of *S. typhi* and *S. paratyphi* A on Wilson and Blair medium. Describe the colony morphology in brief.

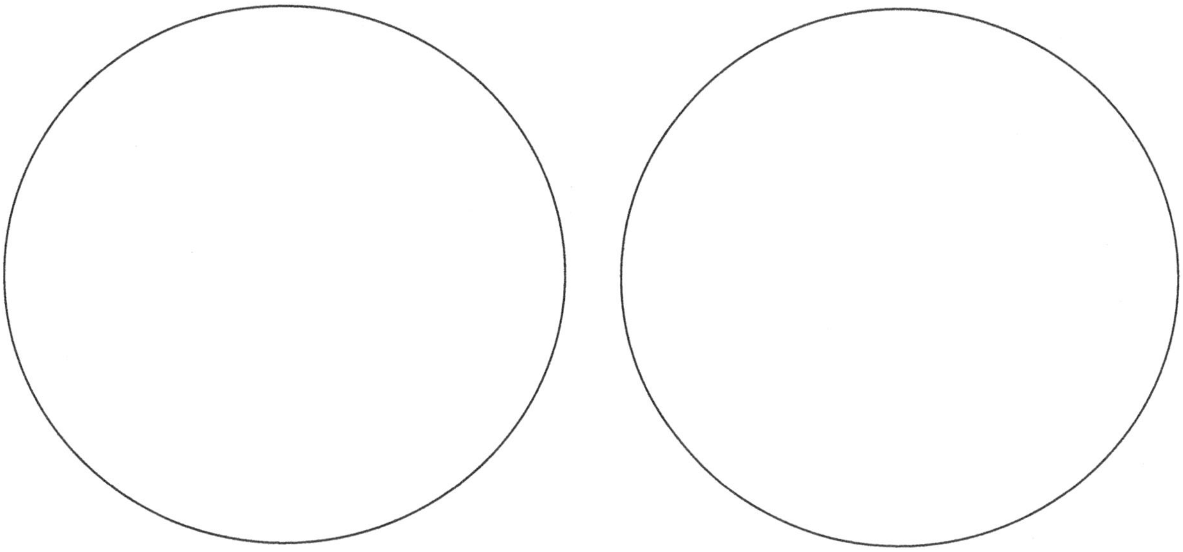

2. Explain the principal, procedure, interpretation, limitation and application of the Widal test.

3. Describe in brief the laboratory diagnosis of food poisoning.

4. Biochemical reaction of *Salmonella* species.

5. A 15-year male presents with complains of Step ladder pyrexia, nausea, malaise and headache since 10 days. On examination there is mild hepatosplenomegaly.

a). What is the probable aetiological agent?

b). How will you arrive at the diagnosis of enteric fever?

6. What are the drugs of choice for therapy?

7. Enumerate the infection caused by Salmonella species.

8. What do you understand by the term Salmonellosis.

Date: ________________

PRACTICAL-20

SHIGELLA

- These are Gram-negative, non-motile, non-sporing and non-capsulated, enterobacteriaceae causing dysentery.
- Dysentery is characterized by the passage of blood stained mucopurulent stools.
- The organisms enter by ingestion and attach themselves to the brush border of the intestinal villi. They multiply within the epithelial cells and spread laterally. They may spread further and multiply in the lamina propria. The infected epithelial cells are destroyed and an inflammatory reaction develops. There is capillary thrombosis and patches of necrotic epithelium are sloughed out.

DEMONSTRATIONS:

A. A Gram's stained smear of *Shigella* species.

B. Growth of *Shigella* on Blood and MacConkey's agar.

PRACTICAL AND EXERCISE:

1. Draw the colony characteristic of *Shigella* A on Wilson and Blair medium. Describe the colony morphology in brief.

2. How will you diagnose a case of *Shigella* dysentery?

3. Classify *Shigella*.

4. Biochemical reaction of *Shigella* species.

Date:________________

PRACTICAL-21

VIBRIO

LEARNING OBJECTIVES:

At the end of the tutorial and practical, the student will be able to

1. Identify the comma shaped bacilli in a specimen of cholera stool stained by Gram's stain and note the paucity of absence of the pus cells.
2. Appreciate the darting motility of V. cholera.
3. Enumerate 3 important biochemical tests for identifying *V. cholera.*
4. List the differences between classical and EI Tor Vibrios.
5. List the non-cholera vibrios and mention the infections produced by them.
6. Mention the principal of cholera red reaction.

INTRODUCTION:

Vibrio are Gram-negative, rigid, curved, rods that are actively motile by means of a polar flagellum. The most important member of the genus of *Vibrio cholerae* the causative agent of cholera.

Cholera is an acute diarrhoeal disease. Frequent passage of fairly large volumes of "rice water" stool, severe dehydration and shock are the characteristics of this illness. Diarrhea is mediated by enterotoxin- an endotoxin secreted by the organism. The clinical severity of the disease may vary. Absence of pus cells and RBCs on the "rice water" stool is a remarkable feature.

Cholera is endemic in the Indian sub-continent and epidemics occur seasonally. The only natural reservoir of V. cholera is man and both convalescent and chronic carriage in man is known. Drinking water contamination by human feces is the main source of infection. Epidemic cholera is associated with fairs, festivals and other large congregations during which sanitary arrangements tend to be unsatisfactory. Other pathogenic members of this genus are NAG (non-agglutinable) Vibrio and V. parahaemolyticus. The NAG Vibrio produce a mild cholera like syndrome and V. parahaemolyticus causes food poisoning associated with marine food.

DEMONSTRATIONS:

1. Smear showing curved Gram-negative bacilli.
2. Hanging drop preparation showing darting motility.
3. Plates of Blood agar and TCBS showing *V. cholerae* colonies.
4. Indole test.
5. Oxidase test.
6. Antibiotic sensitivity plate.
7. Cholera vaccine.
8. Cholera red reaction.
9. String test.
10. Flagellar stain showing polar flagellum.(Optional)

PRACTICAL AND EXERCISE:

Q.1. The important clinical manifestations of cholera are:

Q.2. Which is the most important specimen for the laboratory diagnosis of Cholera?

Q.3. How will you collect a stool specimen for the laboratory diagnosis of Cholera?

Q.4. What is meant by 'darting motility'? How will you demonstrate it?

Q.5. The wet smear examination of rice water stool shows the absence of the following...

Q.6. How will you transport a stool specimen from a suspected case of Cholera to the laboratory at a distant place?

Q.7. Draw a diagram *V. cholerae* seen on Gram stain of freshly passed "rice water" stool?

Q.8. Biochemical Reactions of *V. cholerae*

Q.9. How is *V. cholerae* grown in the laboratory? Mention the important culture media and describe the characters of *V. cholerae* colonies grown on them.

Q.10. Following are the important biochemical tests in the identification of *V. cholerae*....

Q.11. How is the isolate of *V. cholerae* confirmed?

Q.12. Which tests are employed to differentiate V. cholerae from el Tor Vibrio?

Q.13. Mention the recently discovered stain of V. cholerae

Date:________________

PRACTICAL-22

PSEUDOMONAS

LEARNING OBJECTIVES:

At the end of the tutorial and practical, the student will be able to

1. Identify *Pseudomonas aeruginosa* based on their colony characteristics.
2. List the drugs of choice for treating *Pseudomonas* infections.
3. Explain the importance / relevance of infections due to *Pseudomonas*.

INTRODUCTION:

Pseudomonas are Gram-negative, aerobic bacilli that are motile with polar flagella. *Pseudomonas aeruginosa* is the most important species. Natural resistance to variety of anti-microbials is its significant characteristic. It produces a bluish green diffusible pigment. It is an opportunistic pathogen. It is one of the most important bacteria causing nosocomial or Hospital infection.

The metabolism of *Pseudomonas aeruginosa* is oxidative and not fermentative. It therefore shows considerable biochemical inactivity. Positivity of oxidase and citrate tests is noteworthy.

Various typing methods are employed for sub species identification of *Pseudomonas* strains, which helps in epidemiological studies.

DEMONSTRATIONS:

1. Gram stained smear of P. aeruginosa.
2. Culture plates
   a. Nutrient agar with *Pseudomonas aeruginosa* showing diffusible pigment.
   b. NLF colonies of *Pseudomonas aeruginosa* on MacConkey's medium.
3. Hanging drop preparation showing motility of *Pseudomonas aeruginosa.*
4. Oxidase test.
5. Citrate test.
6. Antibiotic sensitivity plate showing multidrug resistance.

PRACTICAL AND EXERCISE:

Q.1. Draw a diagram of *Pseudomonas aeruginosa* as seen on Gram's stain of pus.

Q.2. How will you identify *Pseudomonas aeruginosa*? Mention important cultural characteristics and biochemical reactions.

Q.3. Mention the important infections produced by *Pseudomonas. aeruginosa* in hospitalized patients.

Q.4. Draw antibiotic sensitivity testing of *Pseudomonas. aeruginosa* and interpret it.

Q.5. Biochemical Reactions of *Pseudomonas aeruginosa*

Q.6. Mention the important antibiotics useful in the treatment of *Pseudomonas aeruginosa* infections.

Date:________________

PRACTICAL-23

HOSPITAL ACQUIRED INFECTIONS

LEARNING OBJECTIVES:

At the end of the tutorial and practical, the student will be able to:

1. Define hospital acquired infections.
2. Enumerate the important organisms associated with hospital-acquired infections (HAIs).
3. Enumerate the important areas, high-risk groups for HAIs.
4. List the important tests that will help minimize / eliminate HAIs.
5. List the steps to be taken in case of a respiratory outbreak.

PRACTICAL AND EXERCISE:

Q.1. Define hospital acquired infections.

Q.2. Classify hospital acquired infections.

Q.3. Enlist the following……

a) Organisms responsible for hospital acquired infections

b) Important sources of hospital acquired infection.

c) Routes of spread of pathogens in hospital acquired infection.

Q.4. List the important tests that will help minimize / eliminate HAIs.

Q.5. List the steps to be taken in case of a respiratory outbreak.

Q.6. What do you mean by typing of bacteria? Mention a few important typing methods.

EXTRA SPACE

Date:________________

PRACTICAL-24

YERSINIA

LEARNING OBJECTIVES:

At the end of the tutorial and practical, the student will be able to:

1. Identify *Yersinia pestis* based on its characteristic Gram's stain morphology.
2. Identify rat flea.
3. Explain plague.

INTRODUCTION:

The genus *Yersinia* includes:

1) *Y. pseudotuberculosis* - a primary pathogen of rodents.

2) *Y. enterocolitica,* which causes a primary enteric and systemic disease in animals and man

3) *Y. pestis* - the causative agent of plague.

Plague is a zoonotic disease transmitted from rats to man via the vector' rat flea' (Xenopsylla cheopis). The organisms have a great epidemiological potential but the incidence of plague has dwindled down world over now. Bubonic plague and pneumonic plague are the two main clinical presentations of the disease, both of which can progress to septicaemia. *Y. pestis* are short, stumpy, Gram-negative bacilli, which show characteristic bipolar staining in smear stained with Methylene blue.

Y. pestis grow on ordinary media. The optimum temperature of growth is 27°C. "Stalactite growth" in ghee broth is the noteworthy features of these bacilli.

DEMONSTRATIONS:

1. Methylene blue stained smears of *Y. pestis*.
2. Gram stained smear of brucellae showing the typical coccobacillary forms.
3. Rat flea.
4. Bi-phasic medium.
5. Slide agglutination test with coloured antigen.

PRACTICAL AND EXERCISE:

Q.1. Which samples will you collect from a suspected case of Plague for its laboratory diagnosis?

Q.2. Draw a diagram of *Y. pestis* on Methylene blue staining of direct smear.

Q.3. How will you isolate *Y. pestis* in the laboratory from pathological specimens?

Q.4. Which animal is used in the laboratory diagnosis of plague and why?

Q.5. How will you demonstrate *Y. pestis* infection in rat carcasses?

Q.6. Draw a diagram of rat-flea (Xenopsylla cheopis)

Q.7. Which serological tests are important in the laboratory diagnosis of plague? What is their significance?

Date:________________

PRACTICAL-25

BRUCELLA

LEARNING OBJECTIVES:

At the end of the tutorial and practical, the student will be able to:

1. Define zoonosis
2. Explain serological tests for the laboratory diagnosis of Brucellosis.
3. Culture media required for cultivation of Brucella

INTRODUCTION:

Brucellosis is an important zoonotic disease. Br. abortus from cattle. *Brucella melitensis* from goat and *Brucella suis* from pigs are the principal species. The organisms are very short Gram-negative rods described as coccobacilli. They are capnophilic and grow best on enriched media. They are oxidase positive.

Brucellae infection tends to run a chronic course after the initial acute illness. The organisms are characteristically located intracellularly. A very high index of suspicion is necessary for clinical diagnosis as the clinical picture of Brucellosis is too deceptive.

PRACTICAL AND EXERCISE:

Q.1. Mention the modes of transmission of Brucellae from animals to man.

Q.2. Mention the most important samples collected for the laboratory diagnosis of Brucellosis.

Q.3. Mention the important culture media for the cultivation of Brucellae.

Q.4. What is the important of bi-phasic medium in blood culture for Brucellosis?

Q.5. Mention two important serological tests for the laboratory diagnosis of Brucellosis.

Q.6. Define Zoonosis.

Date:________________

PRACTICAL-26

HAEMOPHILUS

LEARNING OBJECTIVES:

At the end of the tutorial and practical, the student will be able to:

1. Explain satellitism
2. Explain serological tests for the laboratory diagnosis of Brucellosis.
3. Culture media required for cultivation of Brucella

INTRODUCTION:

Haemophilus are small Gram-negative bacilli nutritionally dependent on two factors called factor X (present in haemin) and factor V (coenzyme I &II) found in blood.

H. influenza, H. ducreyi and *H. aegypticus* are the important species. *H. influenza* is a highly pleomorphic bacterium. Both capsulated and non-capsulated strains are found. H. Influenza type b is a commonly encountered pathogen in acute purulent meningitis. It grows on Blood agar, Chocolate agar and media supplemented with factors X and V. The optimum temperature for growth is 37°C and 5 to 10% CO_2 and moisture are helpful for growth. Staphylococcus aureus produces factor V. Therefore colonies of *H. influenzae* growing within 1 to 3 mm of *S. aureus* growth are nutritionally at advantage and larger in size than those colonies of *H. influenzae* growing at a distance. This phenomenon is referred to as "satellitism".

Demonstration of capsular antigen in CSF is very useful in the rapid diagnosis of *H. influenzae* meningitis.

H. ducreyi cause a sexually transmitted ulcerative disease called 'Chancroid'. The organisms are difficult to grow and need enriched media for growth.

H. aegypticus is a causative agent of highly contagious form of conjunctivitis with epidemic potential.

DEMONSTRATIONS:

1. Haemophilus ducreyi smear from a case of chancroid.
2. Gram's stained smear of Haemophilus influenzae showing coco-bacillary and pleomorphic bacilli.
3. West's post-nasal swab.
4. DPT vaccine.
5. DT vaccine.
6. Haemophilus influenza growth on blood agar with Satellitism

PRACTICAL AND EXERCISE:

Q.1. Mention the medically important species of Haemophilus and diseases produced by them.

1. ______________________________
2. ______________________________
3. ______________________________

Q.2. How will you diagnose a case of H. influenzae meningitis?

Q.3. Why should not keep a CSF sample in refrigerator before sending it for culture?

Q.4. Enumerate the rapid diagnostic tests for the diagnosis of meningitis.

Q.5. Which strain of H. influenzae commonly causes meningitis in India?

Q.6. Describe the morphology of H. ducreyi observed in smear prepared from a case of Chancroid.

Q.7. Draw a diagram of Satellitism on blood agar.

Date:________________

PRACTICAL-27

BORDETELLA

LEARNING OBJECTIVES:

At the end of the tutorial and practical, the student will be able to:

1. Explain laboratory diagnosis of whooping cough.
2. Explain prophylaxis of whooping cough.

INTRODUCTION:

Bordetella pertussis and *Bordetella paraperiussis* cause one of the most frequent bacterial respiratory infections in developing countries called 'whooping cough'. The disease is common bellow 5 years of age.

Bordetella pertussis is an Gram-negative, aerobe and grows optimally at 35°C. Bordet-Gengou is a special medium used to cultivate the bacilli on which they produce' bisected pearl' or 'mercury drop' colonies. The patients show marked leucocytosis with relative lymphocytosis. Immunofluorescence staining of smears prepared from postnasal swabs can be used for rapid diagnosis. ELISA test is now a days available for serodiagnosis.

PRACTICAL AND EXERCISE:

Q.1. What is pertussis (whooping cough)?

Q.2. Mention in brief the laboratory diagnosis of whooping cough.

Q.3. Draw a diagram of Bordet-Gengou medium with 'bisected pearl' or 'mercury drop' colonies

Q.4. Mention the prophylaxis of whooping cough.

Date:_______________

PRACTICAL-28

CLOSTRIDIA

LEARNING OBJECTIVES:

At the end of the tutorial and practical, the student will be able to

1. Explain the principle and application of Nagler's test.
2. Enumerate 2 important biochemical tests
3. Differentiate Clostridium welchii and tetani on primary smear examination.
4. Enumerate the different methods of anaerobiosis.
5. Explain how specimens are to be collected and transported in a suspected case of anaerobic infection.
6. Enumerate the media used for cultivating anaerobes.

INTRODUCTION:

The genus Clostridium consists of Gram-positive anaerobic spore forming bacilli. The natural habitat of these organisms is the human and animal intestines, soli, water etc. Gas gangrene, Tetanus and Botulism are the important conditions produced by Clostridia. It is essential to provide anaerobic atmosphere for cultivating Clostridia.

Gas-gangrene:

Wounds, usually the deep penetrating type, contaminated by soil containing spores provide a very good milieu for the growth of Clostridia. The spores develop into vegetative forms and the bacteria grow rapidly. They liberate several potent exotoxins, which lead to necrosis and oedema of the surrounding tissue. The saccharolytic and proteolytic action of the organisms produces large quantity of gas, which adds to the pressure effects of oedema. This causes reduction in the perfusion of the affected part leading to further tissue damage. *Cl. welchii* (*Cl. perfringens*), *Cl. septicum* and *Cl. oedematiens* are the commonest clostridia recovered from gas-gangrene wounds. The disease needs urgent and diligent medical attention. The function of the laboratory here is only to provide confirmation of clinical diagnosis

DEMONSTRATIONS:

1. Gram stained smear of *Cl. welchii*
2. Gram stained smear of *Cl. tetani.*
3. Culture plate showing Nagler reaction.
4. McIntosh Filde's jar.
5. Gas pack or Dynamicro anaerobic jar.
6. Robertson's cooked meat medium.
7. RCM with growth.
8. Stormy clot fermentation.
9. Tetanus toxoid.
10. DTP vaccine.
11. DT vaccine.
12. Anti-tetanus serum.
13. Anti-Gas-gangrene serum.

PRACTICAL AND EXERCISE:

Q.1. Describe morphology of Clostridium welchii

____

____

____

____

Q.2. Enumerate the methods of anaerobiosis.

- ____________________________________
- ____________________________________
- ____________________________________
- ____________________________________
- ____________________________________
- ____________________________________

Q.3. Draw a diagram of McIntosh Fildes' jar and mention briefly how anaerobiosis is produced in the jar.

Q.4. Explain laboratory diagnosis of Gas gangrene

a). Collection of specimens

b). Transportation

c). Gram staining of pus collected from a Gas-gangrene wound.

d). Important media inoculated.

e). Nagler Reaction: Draw a diagram and describe the test procedure.

f). Stormy clot fermentation

TETANUS:

INTRODUCTION:

Tetanus occurs in animals and man when a wound is infected by *Cl. tetani*. The organism is widely distributed in soil and in the intestine of man and animals. Deep puncture wounds, crush injuries etc. especially when contaminated with ionized calcium, soil and other foreign bodies provide very good conditions for multiplication of *Cl. tetani*. The exotoxins; Tetanospasmin secreted by the growing bacilli is transported along the motor neurons to central nervous system. The toxin causes synaptic block of inhibitory control on motor neurons. The disease is characterized by increased muscle tonus and exaggerated muscular response to trivial stimuli leading to violent spasms.

Q.1. Draw a diagram of the smear of *Cl. tetani* demonstrated to you.

Q.2. Important media used for culture of *Clostridium tetani*.

Q.3. Mention the prophylaxis of Tetanus.

BOTULISM:

Botulism is a food born intoxication Meat products like ham, sausage, fish etc. are the important source articles. The organisms are saprophytic and can grow in improperly preserved food. They produce an extremely potent neurotoxin during their growth. The toxin, on consumption along with the food, leads to muscular paralysis through block in production and release of acetylcholine at the neuromuscular junction.

PSEUDOMEMBRANOUS COLITIS:

Pseudomembranous colitis or antibiotic associated colitis is an important condition caused by *Cl. difficile*. Prolonged oral administration of Clindamycin, Lincomycin and some other antibiotics predisposes the disease. The colitis is attributed to selection of drug resistant *Cl. difficile* producing necrotizing toxin, that proliferate in the colon.

Date:________________

PRACTICAL-29

NON-SPORING ANAEROBES

LEARNING OBJECTIVES:

At the end of the tutorial and practical, the student will be able to

1. Explain the Vincent's angina

INTRODUCTION:

Infections due to non-sporing or non-clostridial anaerobes are endogenous in origin. Organisms colonize the mucosal lining of human body. Largest concentration of anaerobes is in colon. However, they colonize oral cavity, nasopharynx, vagina etc. and are present even on skin. When local resistance of the tissue is lowered due to infection, trauma, malignancy or any other reasons the non-sporing anaerobes colonizing the site produce pyogenic infections. Gram-negative bacilli like *Bacteroides*, *Fusobacteria*, Gram-negative cocci like *Veillonella* are the important pathogens encountered in these infections. Non-sporing anaerobes usually produce foul smelling, multimicrobial infections, which are often synergistic with aerobic organisms.

Brain abscess, periodontitis, bronchiectasis, sub-diaphragmatic abscess, appendicitis, pelvic abscess, pyometra, diabetic ulcer infection and septicaemia are the silent examples of anaerobic infection. Metronidazole is a drug of choice in the treatment of non-sporing anaerobic infections.

DEMONSTRATIONS:

1. Gram stained smear of pus from a case of Vincent's angina.
2. Gram stained smear of pus from a case of anaerobic infection showing multimicrobial aetiology.

PRACTICAL AND EXERCISE:

Q.1. Mention two groups of *Bacteroides* found in pyogenic infections.

1. . ____
2. . ____

Q.2. Draw a diagram of Gram stained pus smear from a case of Vincent's angina

Q.3. What are the characteristics of non-clostridial anaerobic infections?

____
____
____
____
____
____
____
____
____
____

Date:________________

PRACTICAL-30

SPIROCHAETES

LEARNING OBJECTIVES:

At the end of the tutorial and practical, the student will be able to

1. Explain the principle and application of Fontana's stain and dark ground illumination.
2. Explain the principle, application, interpretation and limitations of the VDRL test.
3. Recognize the morphological feature of *Treponemes* and *Borrelia.*
4. Enumerate the different tests that can help arrive at the diagnosis of syphilis in its various stages.
5. Explain how specimens are to collected for microscopy from a case of primary syphilis.

INTRODUCTION:

Spirochaetes are long, slender, spiral cells, which show active intrinsic motility but lack flagella. They show rapid lashing movements i.e. sudden flexion and extension of the body, corkscrew like motility and general movement of protoplasm resulting in translatory motion. They vary widely in size and can be 5 to 500 μ long. Larger spirochaetes can be easily seen in stained films but the very thin ones are barely detectable by this method. They are best demonstrated by dark field microscopy in wet preparations.

Spirochaetes belong to the order Spirochaetales that is divided into two families Spirochaetaceae and Treponemataceae. The former includes free-living saprophytic bacteria and the later includes *Treponema, Borrelia* and *Leptospira*, which are pathogenic to man.

TREPONEMA PALLIDUM: This is the causative agent of an important sexually transmitted disease called Syphilis. The organism is 4 to 14 μ long and 0.1 μ thick. It cannot be stained by aniline dyes. It is observed by dark field microscopy and stained by silver impregnation method.

T. pallidum cannot be cultured on artificial culture media.

Syphilis is known to run a very chronic course and shows multisystemic involvement. Involvement of cardiovascular or central nervous system in the late untreated cases is an important characteristic.

DEMONSTRATIONS:

1. A smear stained by Fontana stain showing *T. pallidum*.
2. Gram stained or dilute Carbol Fuchsin stained smear of pus from a case of 'Vincent's Angina'.
3. V.D.R.L. kit.
4. T.P.H.A. kit.
5. V.D.R.L. antigen.
6. Louse.
7. Tick.
8. Guinea pig.
9. FTA test if fluorescent microscope is available.
10. Dark ground microscope (Oral spirochaetes can be demonstrated)

PRACTICAL AND EXERCISE:

Q.1. Draw a smear diagram of *T. pallidum* demonstrated to you. Mention the stain used.

Q.2. Mention two important techniques used for demonstration of *T. pallidum*

Q.3. Enumerate the Syphilitic lesions from which *T. pallidum* can be demonstrated.

Q.4. What does the term VDRL, TRUST and RPR stand for?

Q.5. What do you mean by biological false positive test? (B.F.P)

Q.6. Enumerate the conditions, which give B.F.P. result in V.D.R.L. test.

Q.7. Enumerate the specific tests for serodiagnosis of Syphilis and underline the three most commonly used tests among them.

Q.8. What do you mean by Nichol's strain?

Q.9. What do you mean by Reiter's strain?

Q.10. How do you diagnose neurosyphilis? (Mention a simple serological test)

Q.11. Prophylaxis of Treponema pallidum

BORRELIA

Borrelia are Gram-negative, large, motile, refractile spirochaetes having irregular, wide and open coils. The length is between 10 to 30 μ and breadth between 0.3 to 0.7 μ. They display lashing and rotating movement. Relapsing fever caused by *B. recurrentis*, Vincent's angina (Fuso-spirochaetosis) by *B. vincenti* and Lyme disease by *B. burgdorferi* are the important conditions caused by *Borrelia.*

Q.1. Draw a diagram of pus smear from a case of Vincent's angina.

Q.2. Explain the use of animal inoculation in the laboratory diagnosis of relapsing fever.

LEPTOSPIRA

Leptospira are actively motile, slender Spirochaetes having numerous coils and hooked ends. They are 6 to 20 μ in length and 0.1 μ in thickness. There are several species of *Leptospira* many being saprophytic and a few pathogenic. *Leptospira icterohaemorrhagiae* is a well-known pathogenic species.

The disease leptospirosis varies from mild influenza like illness to severe disease characterized by jaundice, hepatomegaly and haemorrhages called as the Weil's disease. *Leptospira* are the important cause of PUO. The organisms can be demonstrated in wet preparation of centrifuged urine samples or serum samples. Culture is possible from these samples on media enriched with Rabbit serum. The organism can also be grown on chorioallantoic membrane. Serodiagnosis is possible from the end of first week onwards.

Q.1. What are different modes of transmission of Leptospirosis?

Q.2. Enumerate the important samples collected from a patient for the laboratory diagnosis of Leptospirosis?

Q.3. Mention the important methods for demonstration of *Leptospira*.

Q.4. How is Leptospirosis diagnosed serologically?

Date:______________

PRACTICAL-31

ACTINOMYCETES, NOCARDIA

ACTINOMYCETES

LEARNING OBJECTIVES:

At the end of the tutorial and practical, the student will be able to

1. Enumerate the lesions caused by *Actinomycetes*.
2. Identify the Actinomycetes from Gram stained smear of a crushed granule.
3. Describe the laboratory diagnosis of Mycetoma

INTRODUCTION:

Actinomycosis is a chronic granulomatous disease arising endogenously. *Actinomycetes* are true bacteria resembling Fungi in morphology. *A. israelii* is the commonly recovered species. The granulomatous lesions are indurated pointing to skin. The lesions suppurate and form multiple discharging sinuses. The colonies of *Actinomycetes* in the from of 'Sulphur granules' are found in the discharge from the sinuses. The granules are formed of fine Gram-positive mycelia surrounded by a peripheral zone of radiating Gram-negative club shaped structures.

DEMONSTRATIONS:

1. Gram stained smear of a crushed granule from a case Actinomycosis.
2. Culture of *Nocardia*.

PRACTICAL AND EXERCISE:

Q.1. Enumerate the lesions caused by *Actinomycetes*.

____

____

____

____

____

Q.2. How will you demonstrate the causative agent from an Actinomycotic lesion?

Q.3. Draw a diagram of Gram stained smear of the Actinomycotic granule demonstrated to you.

Q.4. How do you culture *Actinomycetes*?

NOCARDIA

Nocardia are Gram-positive, branching bacteria. Some species of *Nocardia* are weakly acid fast. They are obligate aerobes. They grow on simple media but grow slowly. *Nocardia* cause lesions similar to Actinomycosis and systemic infections like pulmonary lesions, which may spread to brain haematogenously.

N. madurae cause Mycetoma; the lesion of foot, popularly known as 'Madura foot'. It is an indurated granulomatous and suppurative infection. It involves sub-cutaneous and deeper tissues like bone. Pus discharge from sinuses may contain granules.

Nocardia from sputum may be confused for tubercle bacilli.

Q.1. Describe the specimen of Mycetoma foot demonstrated to you.

Q.2. Describe the laboratory diagnosis of Mycetoma?

MYCOLOGY

Date:________________

PRACTICAL-32

FUNGI

LEARNING OBJECTIVES:

At the end of the tutorial and practical, the student will be able to

1. Classify fungi
2. Define hyphae, mycelium, spore, conidia.
3. Explain dermatophytosis
4. Explain laboratory diagnosis of fungi

INTRODUCTION:

Fungi are eukaryotic organism with a differentiate nucleus and rigid chitinous cell wall. They lack chlorophyll and hence are saprophytic. Fungi are relatively uncommon cause of disease. Out of a very large number of species known only a few dozen can produce human infections.

A variety of condition leading to immunocompromisation predispose fungal infection e.g. prolonged antibiotic or steroid therapy, malignancies and anticancer chemotherapy or use of radiation, transplantation and its supportive immunosuppressive therapy, uncontrolled diabetes mellitus, nutritional deficiencies, Acquired Immune Deficiency Syndrome (AIDS) etc. With the surging AIDS pandemic fungal infections are encountered more frequently now days.

For the purpose of convenience the fungal infections are classified as superficial mycosis and deep or systemic mycosis. The fungal infections of skin, hair and nail are usually caused by dermatophytes and are milder variety of infection. On the other hand, 'deep mycosis' often leads to systemic involvement and if not managed properly may lead to fatality.

Sabouraud's Dextrose Agar (SDA) is a commonly employed for the cultivation of fungi. Most of the fungi produce long branching filaments called hyphae. The hyphae may be septate or non-septate. Some fungi do not form mycelia and are called 'Yeast'. 10% KOH mount is commonly used to diagnose superficial mycosis. Some stains used for fungi are Lactophenol cotton blue, Mayer's mucicarmin, Periodic Acid Schiff (PAS) etc.

DEMONSTRATIONS:

1. Sabouraud's Agar-plain.
2. Sabouraud's Agar with growth.
3. SDA showing pigmentation on the obverse side.
4. SDA showing pigmentation on the reverse side.
5. Gram stained smear of *Candida albicans*.
6. Germ tube test.
7. LCB mount of available fungi to show microconidia, macroconidia and hyphae.
8. *Cryptococcus* with negative stain.

PRACTICAL AND EXERCISE:

Q.1. What are the different ways to classify fungi?

Q.2. Define the following-

- Hyphae

____

____

- Mycelium

____

____

Spores

____

____

Conidia

____

____

Q.3. What are the different types of spores?

____

____

____

____

____

____

____

____

____

____

____

____

____

____

Q.4. What do you mean by dimorphic fungi? Give examples.

Q.5. Draw and label the diagrams of slides demonstrated to you-

KHO preparation of skin scraping

Macroconidia of Trichophyton

Macroconidia of Epidermophyton

Macroconidia of Microsporum

***Cryptococcus neoformans* (Negative Stain)**

Gram stained smear of *Candida albicans*.

Germ tube test

Rhinosporidiosis

Aspergillosis

Penicillium

Mucor

Rhizopus

Q.6. How will you diagnose a case of dermatophytosis?

Q.7. How will you diagnose a case of Cryptococcal meningitis?

Q.8. Enumerate some fungi, which cause deep mycosis.

Q.9. Which fungal infections are strongly associated with "HIV infection'?

VIROLOGY

Date:________________

PRACTICAL-33

GENERAL PROPERTIES OF VIRUSES

LEARNING OBJECTIVES:

At the end of the tutorial and practical, the student will be able to:

1. Define a virus.
2. Enumerate important DNA and RNA viruses and infection caused by them.
3. Enumerate the different methods for demonstration and cultivation of viruses.
4. Explain the limitations of light microscopy for direct demonstration.
5. Recognize uninfected cell lines.
6. Recognize inclusions of Negri bodies and Molluscum contagiosum.
7. Enumerate the uses of tissue culture bottle.
8. Enumerate the various routes of inoculation on embryonated egg and the application of each route.
9. Describe the growth on chorioallantoic membrane.
10. Enumerate the different cytopathic effects produced by viral growth.
11. Explain the different steps involved in the laboratory diagnosis of viral infection.
12. Enumerate the viral infections for which antiviral drugs are available.

INTRODUCTION:

Viruses are ultramicroscopic, metabolically inert, obligate intracellular parasites which contain either DNA or RNA but never both.

The laboratory diagnosis of viral infection involves

a) Direct demonstration of the virus or viral antigens or viral nucleic acid (PCR)

By using light microscope (inclusion bodies), electron microscope of fluorescent microscope.

b) Isolation of viruses in tissue culture, embryonated eggs or laboratory animals.

c) Serological tests for demonstrating significant antibody titres.

DEMONSTRATIONS:

1. Section of brain showing Negri bodies
2. Section of skin showing inclusions of Molluscum contagiosum
3. Slide of cell line
4. Chorioallantoic membrane with growth.
5. Tissue culture bottle with cell line. (optional)
6. Leighton's tube
7. Polio vaccine
8. Haemagglutination test
9. ELISA for HIV infection.

PRACTICAL AND EXERCISE:

1. Draw the diagrams of the tissue culture bottle and Leighton's tube demonstrated.

2. Draw the diagrams of Cell line, Negri bodies and Molluscum slides.

3. Draw a well labeled diagram of the various routes of inoculation on embryonated eggs.

4. Enumerate laboratory tests for detection of antibodies against HIV infection.

5. What are the applications of haemagglutination and haemagglutination inhibition tests in viral diseases.

6. Write a brief note on Universal Precautions.

____

____

____

____

____

____

____

____

____

____

____

____

____

____

7. Enumerate 4 DNA viruses and 4 RNA viruses and mention the infection produced by them.

DNA Viruses: 1.____

2.____

3.____

4.____

RNA Viruses: 1.____

2.____

3.____

4.____

8.Enumerate 4 congenital viral infections.

1.____

2.____

3.____

4.____

PARASITOLOGY

PARASITOLOGY

LEARNING OBJECTIVES:

At the end of the tutorial and practical, the student will be able to

1. Enumerate the different parasites causing human infections.
2. Classify the parasites.
3. Describe the morphology of the important stages of the parasite seen in human beings.
4. Explain the life cycle of the parasites.
5. Explain the pathogenesis and laboratory diagnosis of parasitic infections.
6. Enumerate the differences between the various classes of parasites.
7. Enumerate the drug of choice for a given parasitic infection.
8. Perform faeces examination, both saline and iodine mount and interpret the findings.
9. Identify correctly under the microscope the different stages of the various intestinal and tissue parasites.
10. Identify the different cellular elements in stool specimen under the microscope.
11. Identify plasmodia, trypanosomal and filarial parasite on peripheral blood smear.
12. Identify the tissue section of cestodes.
13. Identify the tissue section of adult filarial worm.
14. Identify *Toxoplasma.*
15. Identify the adult worms of cestodes, trematodes and nematodes.
16. Identify correctly the vectors transmitting parasitic infections.

INTRODUCTION:

Parasitology is the study of parasites and host-parasite relationship. The term 'parasite' is restricted here, to parasites of the animal kingdom. The animal parasites of man belong to three phyla-

1. Phylum protozoa,
2. Phylum platyhelminthes and
3. Phylum nemathelminthes.

Phylum as you may recall; is divided into classes, orders, families, genera and species. The name of a parasite always shows its genus and species. The systematic study of a parasite involves the knowledge of geographical distribution, habitat, morphology, life cycle, modes of infection (sources of infection, portals of entry means used to seek entry) and their pathogenic effects, Further, to complete the study, laboratory diagnosis of infection, treatment, prophylactic measures against infection are also essential.

SOME COMMON PROTOZOA:

Protozoa are unicellular organisms consisting of a nucleus and cytoplasm. According to their habitat the protozoa fall into three groups:

1. Intestinal protozoa
2. Atrial protozoa living in mouth, vagina and urethra and
3. Blood protozoa living in blood or blood forming organs.

Zoologically, the phylum Protozoa is divided into four classes:

1. Rhizopoda,
2. Ciliata,
3. Sporozoa &
4. Mastigophora.

RHIZOPODA:

Pseudopodia are the organs of locomotion in Rhizopoda, *Entamoeba histolytica* (*Entamoeba*= genus: *histolytica*= species) is the only pathogenic species. The non-pathogenic species include *E. coli*, *Endolimax nana*, *lodamoeba butschli*, *Dientamoeba fragilis* (all intestinal) and *E. gingivals* (atrial).

CILIATA:

The protozoa of this class move by means of cilia. *Balantidium coli* is the only species pathogenic to man, causing dysentery. It is a common intestinal ciliate of pigs, which serves as a reservoir of infection. Man is infected by swallowing the cysts of *B. coli* in food contaminated by pig faecal material, or through hands soiled by handling pigs.

SPOROZOA:

Following parasites of this class are pathogenic to man. The malarial parasite, a blood protozoan, is responsible for malaria. *Cryptosporidium*, *lsospora hominis* and Microsporidia are intestinal protozoa causing diarrhoea especially in immunosuppressed individuals. *Toxoplasma* inhabits the tissues and causes a systemic disease. Parasites of this class do not have any organ of locomotion. They have alternation of generation with alternation of host. Sexual reproduction leads to formation of sporozoites.

MASTIGOPHORA:

These organisms have characteristic shape and possess one or more flagella, which are organs of locomotion. They inhabit the gastrointestinal tract (GIT), e.g. *Giardia*; genitourinary tract, e.g. *Trichomonas*; or the blood-e.g. *Leishmania*.

Date:_______________

PRACTICAL-34

PROTOZOA-I

INTESTINAL PROTOZOA

***Entamoeba histolytica*:** It exists in two forms. The vegetative from – the trophozoite and the resting resistant form – the cyst. Cyst is the infective form. When ingested, the cyst wall ruptures in the small intestine and daughter amoebae are released. They are invasive and cause amoebic colitis. The acute form is called as acute amoebic dysentery, which is characterized by passage of loose motions mixed with blood and mucous. The infection can persist at a low level causing chronic intestinal amoebiasis. If trophozoites enter the portal circulation, they can lodge in different organs causing extra-intestinal amoebiasis, commonly diffuse amoebic hepatitis or liver abscess.

Laboratory diagnosis:

1. Intestinal amoebiasis – Diagnosis rests on examination of freshly passed stools.
   - Amoebic dysentery – Trophozoites detected in saline mount.
   - Chronic amoebiasis – Cysts detected in iodine mount.
2. Extra-intestinal amoebiasis – Detection of antibodies to *E. histolytica* in patient's serum by using different serologic tests e.g. IHA, CFT, ELISA etc.

***Giardia lamblia*:** This is a flagellate existing in trophozoite and cyst form. The trophozoite attaches itself to jejunal mucosa and prevents absorption of fats. It leads to steatorrhea and malabsorption syndrome. The infection is common in children.

Laboratory diagnosis: It involves examination of fresh stool specimen. Actively motile trophozoites are seen in the stools in acute disease while the iodine mount shows typical cysts in the chronic form of the disease.

***Entamoeba coli*:** It is a nonpathogenic amoeba seen in stools of healthy individuals. It must be differentiated from the pathogenic one.

***Cryptosporidium*:** This is an opportunistic pathogen. It causes disease in cattle and also causes self-limiting diarrhoea in normal healthy individuals. It can cause fatal diarrhoea in immunocompromised individuals and is commonly found in association with AIDS patients.

The disease can be diagnosed by detection of *Cryptosporidium* oocysts in a smear of stool stained with modified Ziehl-Neelsen (ZN) stain (Kiniyon stain). They are 7-9 µ in size, round in shape and acid fast.

***Isospora belli*:** This is also an opportunistic parasite common in AIDS patients where it causes fatal diarrhoea. It is also acid fast, spindle shaped with two sporocysts inside. The size is 25 µ × 15 µ.

DEMONSTRATIONS:

1. A drawing showing microscopic appearance of saline mount of stool in acute amoebic dysentery. The fresh specimens may be available in the side laboratory of words or in the OPD laboratory. Note the typical appearance of the trophozoite and various components of the dysenteric stool
2. An iodine mount of stool from a patient with chronic amoebiasis showing cysts of *E. histolytica*. Note presence of 1 to 4 nuclei and the glycogen mass.
3. An iodine mount of stool from a healthy individual showing cysts of *E. coli.* Note the large size and presence of 4-8 nuclei.
4. Drawing of a trophozoite of *Giardia lamblia.*
5. An iodine mount of stool from a patient of chronic giardiasis showing cysts of *Giardia.*
6. A smear of stool of an AIDS patient stained with modified ZN stain showing acid fast rounded oocysts of *Cryptosporidium* (5-7 µ in size).
7. A smear of stool of an AIDS patient stained with modified ZN stain showing acid fast spindle shaped oocysts of *Isospora* (optional)
8. Large intestine –specimen of acute dysentery showing amoebic ulcers with undermined edges and the intervening normal mucosa.
9. Large intestine–specimen of amoebic colitis. Note the thickening and loss of rugosity of mucosa.
10. Liver - Amoebic abscess. Note the abscess cavity with shaggy necrotic wall.

PRACTICAL AND EXERCISE:

- Prepare saline and iodine mount of the stool sample provided to you.
- Observe the cysts of *E. histolytica* and *Giardia lamblia.*

1. Write the laboratory diagnosis of acute amoebic dysentery.

2. Write the differences between amoebic dysentery and bacillary dysentery.

3. Draw diagrams of all the slides demonstrated to you.

Trophozoite of *E. histolytica*
(Saline mount)

Cysts of *E. histolytica*
(Iodine mount)

Appearance of stool in acute amoebic dysentery

Trophozoite of *E. coli*

Cyst of *E. coli*

***Giardia* trophozoite**

***Giardia* cyst**

***Cryptosporidium*-modified ZN stain**

***Isospora*-modified ZN stain**

Date:________________

PRACTICAL-35

PROTOZOA-II

BLOOD AND TISSUE PROTOZOA

In this practical you will be studying *Plasmodium* and *Toxoplasma*, i.e. the Sporozoa causing blood and tissue infection.

Plasmodium: There are four species causing infection in man - *P. vivax, P. falciparum, P. malariae,* and *P. ovale*. Of these, the former two are common. They are transmitted to man by mosquito bite. They cause malaria.

P. vivax	-	benign tertian malaria
P. falciparum	-	malignant tertian malaria
P. malariae	-	quatrain malaria
P. ovale	-	ovale tertian malaria

Life cycle: It consists of two stages

1. The sexual stage in mosquito (i.e. the completion of gametogony and sporogony)and
2. The asexual stage in man (the schizogony and beginning of gametogony).

In man the parasite resides mainly in RBCs, undergoes schizogony and causes repeated destruction of RBCs. The RBCs rupture leading to liberation of merozoites, which coincides with the malarial paroxysm. The periodicity of malarial attack depends on duration of schizogony and hence differs in different species of plasmodia. It is 48 hours for all the three others except *P. malariae* where it is 72 hours. The disease involves organs of reticuloendothelial system which undergo hyperplasia and they are infiltrated with parasitized RBCs. Spleen, bone marrow, brain are the commonly affected organs, spleen being affected the most.

Falciparum malaria causes serious complications like pernicious malaria due to parasitization of large number of RBCs and sequestration of parasitized cells in internal organ capillaries. This leads to blockade of capillaries. If capillaries of CNS are affected, this can lead to convulsions, paralysis, coma and death.

Laboratory diagnosis: It rests mainly on examination of peripheral blood smear (PBS) after Leishman's or Giemsa staining. 'Thick smear' is used rapid diagnosis while 'thin smear' is used for species identification. In case of *P. vivax*, *P. malariae* and *P. ovale* all erythrocytic forms are seen in PBS while in *P. falciparum* only the rings or the gametocytes are seen.

***Toxoplasma gondii*:** This protozoan parasite is normally present in intestine of cat and in tissues of different animals like goat, sheep, chicken etc. It is transmitted to man by ingestion, inhalation, or inoculation. Cat faces and raw or undercooked meat are common sources of infection. In the intestinal epitheliums, it undergoes the enterohepatic cycle and the infective oocysts are released in the feces. Entry of organisms by other routes leads to formation of tissue cysts, which get lodged in different tissues. In most of the individuals, the infection is asymptomatic but in about 20% patients, it can cause hepatosplenomegaly, lymphadenopathy, skin rash, pneumonitis, myocarditis or encephalomyelitis. Infection of a pregnant mother can lead to congenital infection of the fetus, causing mainly cerebral calcifications, microcephaly, mental retardation, chorioretinitis, etc. It can also cause abortions and stillbirths. CNS toxoplasmosis in an AIDS patient is many times fatal.

The diagnosis is achieved by antibody detection or by tissue biopsy in which the tissue cysts are detected.

DEMONSTRATIONS:

1. Peripheral blood smear showing ring from of *P. vivax*. Note large size of ring, the red nucleus and blue ring. Also note that the parasitized RBC is larger than non-parasitized RBCs.
2. Peripheral blood smear showing amoeboid from of *P. vivax*. Note presence of Schuffner's granules and large size of RBC.
3. Peripheral blood smears showing a schizont of *P. vivax*. The merozoites are arranged in a rosette around the central mass of pigment.

4. Peripheral blood smears showing the ring form *P. falciparum*. The rings are small and more than one ring are present in the RBCs. Accole forms may be seen. The RBC size is normal.
5. Peripheral blood smears showing gametocytes of *P. falciparum* and *P. vivax*. Note the difference in the size and shape.
6. Section of brain in cerebral malaria - The capillaries are congested and filled with parasitized RBCs.
7. A drawing/picture/slide showing tissue forms of *T. gondii*.

PRACTICAL AND EXERCISE:

1. How and when the peripheral blood smear is collected and prepared for laboratory diagnosis of malaria?

2. Mention important serodiagnositc tests for toxoplasmosis.

3. How to prepare thick and thin smear. Describe the procedure of staining.

4. Answer following questions in brief.

a) Name the species of malarial parasites causing human infection. Which one of these can cause serious complication?

b) What is Blackwater fever?

5. Draw the different forms of malarial parasite found in peripheral blood and describe in brief

EXTRA SPACE

Date:________________

PRACTICAL-36

PROTOZOA-III

HAEMOFLAGELLATES & TISSUE FLAGELLATES

This group includes two genera – *Leishmania* and *Trypanosoma*. These organisms are present in blood, tissues and body fluids. They are transmitted to man by vector bite.

Leishmania- These are monoflagellate protozoa affecting the reticuloendothelial system (RES). There are three important species-

L. donovani – causes visceral leishmaniasis.

L. tropica – causes oriental sore.

L. brasiliensis – causes Espundia.

The vector is sandfly. The parasite exists in two forms – The amastigote form in human tissues and the promastigote form in sand fly and culture medium. As the main site of affection is the reticuloendothelial system (RES). The amastigote form is present in cells of RES and is called as LD bodies.

Laboratory diagnosis:

It rests on:

1. Demonstration of parasites in clinical samples like bone marrow or splenic aspirate or
2. Isolation i.e. culture &
3. Serology – Demonstration of specific and nonspecific antibodies using non-leishmanial and leishmanial antigens.

***Trypanosoma*:** The vector for transmission is Tsetse fly and reduviid bug. Three species are pathogenic to man, *T. gambiense* and *T. rhodesiense* cause African sleeping sickness and *T. cruzi* causes Chagas' disease. The natural reservoirs are antelopes an (*T. gambiense* and *T. rhodesiense*) and armadillos and probably cats and dogs (*T. cruzi*).

The organisms are morphologically indistinguishable. Human tryanosomiasis is not found in India.

Laboratory diagnosis: Rests on –

1. Demonstration of parasite in- i) peripheral blood smear stained by Leishman's or Giemsa stain & ii) in CSF
2. Culture on Novy-MacNeal-Nicolle (NNN) medium,
3. Demonstration of specific antigen and antibody in patient's serum and CSF.

Trichomonas vaginalis: This is genitourinary parasite existing only in trophozoite form. It is pear shaped organism with one large nucleus, four flagella a cytostome. The cytoplasm is granular. The organism is actively motile.

It causes one of the commonest sexually transmitted disease- Trichomoniasis. It causes vaginitis and urethritis in females and urethritis and prostatitis in males. In females, the disease is characterized by foul smelling vaginal discharge and severe vulval pruritus. In males it may be asymptomatic.

Laboratory diagnosis: Demonstration of the motile parasite in wet mount of vaginal secretions and urine or centrifuged deposit of urine.

DEMONSTRATIONS:

1. A smear of bone marrow from a case of Kala-azar stained with Leishman's stain showing LD bodies within the macrophages. They are small, oval, 2 μ in size, a red stained nucleus and a kinetoplast lying at right angles to the nucleus.
2. A smear of splenic aspirate from a case of Kala-azar stained with Leishman's stain showing the macrophages containing LD bodies.
3. A smear of liver showing LD bodies in Kupffer cells.
4. A smear from culture on NNN medium – Leishman's stain – shows promastigote forms of Leishmania. They are elongated, fusiform with a red central nucleus, blue cytoplasm, red stained basal body a flagellum. Undulating membrane is absent.
5. Sandy fly, it is laterally flattened has pairs of wings, and legs and or proboscis.

6. A smear from oriental sore – Leishman's stain –shows *L. tropica*. They are very similar to *L. donovani*.
7. A smear of peripheral blood from a case of sleeping sickness – Leishman's stain – shows *T. gambiense*. Fusiform organism about 15-40 μ in size. Nucleus is central. Kinetoplast is at the posterior end. Flagellum arises from it, runs along the outer border of undulating membrane and continues as flagellum beyond the anterior end.
8. A wet mount of vaginal discharge from a case of Trichomoniasis. See the actively motile *T. vaginalis*.
9. A PAS stained smear of vaginal discharge, showing *T. vaginalis*, See the typical pear shape, flagella, cytostome, and the pointed tip of axoneme coming out at the posterior end.

PRACTICAL AND EXERCISE:

Outline laboratory diagnosis of Kala-azar.

Answer following question in brief.

1. Name the different species of *Leishmania* and mention the diseases caused by them.

2. Name the sexually transmitted disease caused by a "Protozoal" parasites.

3. What is the pathogenicity *Trypanosoma gambiense* ?

DEMONSTRATIONS:

Date:________________

PRACTICAL-36

HELMINTHES

The multicellular parasitic worms are called as 'Helminthes'. They belong to two phyla

- Phylum Platyhelminthes-flat worms.
- Phylum Nemathelminthes-round worms.

Platyhelminthes are further classified into two classes

- Cestodes – Tape worms
- Trematodes – Flukes

CESTODES:

These are ribbon like flat worms with long segmented body. The body consists of scolex (head), neck and strobila (body). The body is composed of proglottides (segments). These worms are hermaphrodites. The eggs are released in feces of definitive host while larval form is present in tissues of intermediate host.

The human infections are caused by:

1. *Taenia saginata* (beef tapeworm)
2. *Taenia solium* (pork tapeworm)
3. *Echinococcus granulosus* (hydatid worm)
4. *Hymenolepis nana* (dwarf tapeworm)
5. *Diphyllobothrium latum* (fish tape worm)

These worms pass their life cycle in 2 or 3 hosts. The adults are present in small intestine of definitive host and eggs passed in feces. The intermediate hosts are infected via food contaminated with feces containing eggs. The embryo is released in stomach; it penetrates the mucosa, enters circulation and lodges in tissues of host. There, it develops into larval form. Eating infected tissues of the intermediate host infects the definitive host. Now the larva develops into adult worm, which attaches itself to mucosa of small intestine, matures and the cycle repeats.

Sr. No.	Name	Morphology	Definitive Host	Inter-mediate Host	Larval form	Pathogenicity	Laboratory Diagnosis
1	*T. saginata*	Adult 5-10 mtrs. Segment.>1000 Scolex-4 suckers No rostellum	Man	Cattle	Cysticercus bovis	GIT disturbance	Stool exam for eggs, segments
2	*T. solium*	Adult 2-3 mtrs. Segments 500-1000 Scolex with 4 suckers rostellum with double row of hooklets globular	Man	Pig	Cysticercus cellulosae	GIT disturbance Cysticercosis of various organs	Stool exam. for eggs segments, Serology
3	*H. nana*	Adult 1-4 cm Segments upto 200 Scolex-small globular with rostellum and hooklets	Man Rodents, Mice & Rats	Absent	Cysticercoid s	Abdominal pain & diarrhoea in severe infection	Stool exam eggs.
4	*E. granulosus*	Adult 3-6 mm Scolex-small with rostellum and hooklets	Canines Dogs, Fox, Wolves	Man Sheep, Cattle	Hydatid cyst	Hydatid cyst in liver, lung, bone, spleen, etc.	Casoni's test

DEMONSTRATIONS:

1. A complete tapeworm (*T. saginata*). Note the globular head and the large number of proglottides.
2. A scolex of *T. saginata* showing four round suckers: The head is bald. Contrast this appearance with that of *T. solium* shown in 6.
3. A mature gravid segment of *T. saginata*: Its length is more than its breadth and shows a large number of compound lateral branches (more than 15) of the central uterine stem.
4. An ovum of *T. saginata* (or *solium*): the egg is round (30 to 45 mm) with a thick, striated, brown embryophore and an oncosphere with six hooklets (hexacanth embroyo). Ova of *T. saginata* and *T. solium* cannot be differentiated from one another.
5. Cysticercus cellulosae: This is the larval stage of *T. solium* found in the striated muscle of the intermediate host (pigs). It consists of a small cyst (10x3 mm) with an invaginated

scolex. Cysticercus bovis occurring in cattle is the larval form of *saginata* and is identical in appearance.

6. A scolex of *T. solium*: shows besides suckers, a finger like projection at its anterior end (called rostellum) which bears a double row of hooklets.
7. A mature, gravid segment of *T. solium*; shows few compound lateral branches of the central uterine stem. The size and shape are similar to those of *T. saginata.*
8. An ovum of *H. nana* shows the eggshell. The embryophore is filled with thread-like filament.
9. A specimen of the liver showing a hydatid cyst.
10. A deposit of hydatid fluid (hydatid sand) shows invaginated scolices with hooklets.
11. A section of hydatid cyst. Note the three layers of the cyst wall, the germinal epithelium and presence of brood capsules.

PRACTICALS AND EXERCISES:

1. Draw all demonstration slides.

2. Examine the given stool sample for presence of cestode of ova. Note the findings.

Scolex- *T. saginata*

Scolex- *T. solium*

Egg of Taenia

Gravid segment- *T. saginata*

Gravid segment *T. solium*

Egg of *H. nana*

Cysticercus cellulosae **Hydatid sand** **Hydatid cyst wall**

Date:________________

PRACTICAL-38

TREMATODES

INTRODUCTION:

Trematodes are flat leaf like worms having a body with holes i.e. the acetabula are present.

CHARACTERISTICS:

- Unsegmented mostly flat leaf like worms except Schistosomiasis.
- Attached to their host by means of suckers.
- No body cavity.
- Digestive system incomplete.
- They are hermaphrodites except Schistosomes.
- Most trematodes eggs are operculated (with lids).

The important species causing human infections are: *S. haematobium, S. mansoni, S. japonicum*.

LIFE CYCLE:

- The adult worms reside at various sites in human beings.
- The eggs are passed in urine or faeces.
- The egg contains a fully formed miracidium which hatches out when it comes in contact with water. The miracidium swims actively and penetrates an appropriate snail host.
- After entry into a snail it changes into a aporocyst and finally a cercariae.
- The cercariae emerge from the snail mainly on exposure to light and penetrate appropriate animal host.
- The parasite is transformed to shistosomula in the animal host.
- The schistosolmula first enters the systemic circulation, the portal circulation and mature in the mesenteric veins and vesical plexus depending upon the species.
- The pathology is due to the host reaction to the eggs.

DEMONSTRATIONS:

1. The eggs of *Schistosoma haematobium* and *Schistosoma mansoni.*
2. Adult Schistosomes
3. Intermediate host (snail)
4. *Fasciola hepatica*

PRACTICAL AND EXERCISE:

1. Describe in brief the laboratory diagnosis of *S. haematobium* infections.

2. Draw the microscopic picture of the eggs of the various Schistosomes.

3. Draw the adult worms of *S. haematobium* and *Fasciola hepatica*.

Date:______________

PRACTICAL-39

NEMATHELMINTHES: INTESTINAL NEMATODES

Nemathelminthes or roundworms are unsegmented worms with a complete digestive tract. The sexes are separate. The parasitic species belong to the class Nematoda. According to the habitat of the adult parasites, the nematodes can be divided into:

1. Intestinal nematodes, which live in the lumen of the small intestine or buried in the mucosa; these are *Necator americanus* and *Ancylostoma duodenale* (hookworms) *Necator* being the most commonly found parasite of the two; in India. *Ascaris lumbricoides*, *Strongyloides stercoralis*, *Trichuris trichiura* and *Trichinella spiralis* are the other important parasites in this group. One species, *Enterobius vermicularis*, lives in the caecum and appendix.
2. Somatic or tissue nematodes, which live in the subcutaneous tissue (*Onchocerca volvulus*, *Loa loa* and *Dracunculus medinensis*) or lymphatics (*Wuchereria bancrofti* and *Brugia malayi*).

INTESTINAL NEMATODES: GENERAL CONSIDERATIONS

The stages in the life history of these are: adult worm, egg, rhabditiform larva and filariform larva. A rhabditiform larva has a short esophagus and an open mouth, it is the non-infective, first stage larva. A filariform larva nematodes has long esophagus and closed mouth, it is the non-feeding, infective, second stage larva. Intestinal do not require intermediate hosts. Eggs in various stages of development (in oviparous worms) or first stage larvae (in viviparous worms) are passed in feces and they mature into infective larvae either within the eggshell or outside the host body, usually on soil. The infective larvae either penetrate the skin of the host (as happens in the case of hookworms and *S. stercoralis*) or the eggs with hatched larvae are swallowed. *T. spiralis* is the exception in that the larvae are liberated in the blood vessels of the intestinal mucosa by the female from there they are carried to muscles to develop into the infective form. In case of *Enterobius vermicularis*, the ova are deposited on the perianal skin by the female and are rarely passed in the feces.

HOOKWORMS:

Necator americanus and *Ancylostoma duodenale* are the species infecting man. These are small worms 8-12 mm in length. With the anterior extremity slightly bent to form a hook. It is a very commonly encountered worm in our country. The adults attach themselves firmly to the mucosa of the small intestine and feed on blood. When passed in feces the eggs are in various stages of development. Further development takes place in soil; rhabditiform larvae hatch out of egg and moults to form filariform larvae. The latter is infective and penetrates the skin. Entering the venous stream the larvae are carried to the right side of the heart and through the pulmonary artery, to the capillaries of the lung. Here they erode the capillaries and enter into the alveolar lumen. Migrating up the respiratory tract and epiglottis they are swallowed and come to the esophagus, pass down into the small intestine and develop into adults.

The clinical manifestations of hookworm infection consist of dermatitis at the site of entry (ground itch) and pneumonitis during larval migration through the lungs. The worms produce a severe anaemia, usually a microcytic hypochromic type.

Ascaris lumbricoides (roundworm):

Adult male worm is little smaller than female, it measures 15-30 cm × 2-4 mm. adult female worm is larger than male, it measures 20-40 cm × 3-6 mm. Ascariasis is a widespread infection especially in children. The adult worms live in the lumen of the small intestine. Eggs are passed in feces. Larvae develop inside the eggs lying on soil. When these are swallowed, the embryo comes out of the thick eggshell in the small intestine. It pierces the mucosa and via blood vessels reaches the liver and is carried to the right side of the heart and lungs. Here it leaves the blood stream to gain entry into the lumen of the alveoli and then crawls up the bronchi and trachea to the pancreatic ducts. Presence of larvae in the alveolar sacs sometimes produces pneumonitis.

Strongyloides stercoralis:

This measures only 1 to 2 cm. the adult male has a transient existence. The adult female lives buried in the mucosa of the small intestine. Eggs are passed in feces. Larvae develop inside the eggs lying on soil. When these are swallowed, the embryo comes out of the thick eggshell in the small intestine. It pierces the mucosa and enters blood vassels. Here it leaves the blood stream to gain entry into the lumen of the alveoli and then crawls up the bronchi and trachea to the epiglottis. It is swallowed and carried into the small intestine, again, to develop into an adult.

The presence of adults in the small intestine may not cause symptoms, or may cause abdominal discomfort and colicky pain. In children masses of entangled worms may cause intestinal obstruction. Migrating worms may lay eggs in the tissue. These hatch rhabditiform larvae come out into the lumen of the small intestine to be passed in the feces. On soil, these develop into filariform larvae, the infective forms, which penetrate the human skin. The further life cycle is like that of hookworms. In addition, parasite is also capable of free existence in moist soil. This cycle is as follows: rhabditiform larvae to adult males and females to mating ova to rhabditiform larvae. Filariform larvae are also produced and are a potential source of infection for man.

Adults may cause mucous diarrhoea: pneumonitis and dermatitis may occur during migration of the larvae.

Trichuris trichiura (whipworm):

Infection by this worm is very common. The adult worms measures 4-5 cm and in general appearance resembles a whip. The worm has a long thin cord-like anterior and short stout posterior portion. The female is slightly larger. The posterior end of the female is rounded whereas that of the male is curved and bears as spicule. The adults are found in the caecum, ileum, appendix and colon, the anterior portion (which is really the esophagus) being buried in the mucosa. The worm lays eggs, which are passed in the feces. Larvae hatch within the eggs in water or soil. Infection occurs when such eggs are swallowed. The intestinal juices dissolve the eggshell and the liberated larvae directly mature into adults.

The infection produces mild gastro-intestinal disturbances and vague abdominal pain. Examining feces for eggs makes the laboratory diagnosis.

Enterobius vermicularis (thread worm):

This infection is very common in children. The adult worms live in the caecum. The male worm has a short life and dies after fertilizing the female. The gravid female crawls down the large intestine and work its way out of the anus during the night hours. The eggs containing larvae are deposited on the perianal skin and are infective. Infection is acquired by swallowing eggs that contaminate the fingers and underclothing. Autoinfection is very common. Larvae from the swallowed eggs directly develop into adult females and males in the intestine.

The infection may be symptomless but usually there is pruritus. It may be a cause of nocturnal enuresis in children. The diagnosis is made by recovering eggs from the perianal region by means of cellophane or cellulose tape and swabs, the swabbing being done before a stool is passed and before a bath. The parasite can often be seen in the feces after a strong saline purgative.

Trichinella spiralis:

The infection is restricted to pork-eating people. It is very uncommon in our country. The adult worm is a parasite of rats, pigs, other carnivorous animals and man. The male worm is half the size of the female. It has a short life and dies after fertilizing the female. The female measures 3 mm × 60 mm. the gravid female (viviparous) liberates larvae, which find their way into blood vessels and lymphatics, and are carried into various organs of same host (heart, brain, lung, liver, kidneys and skeletal muscle). Thus, the same host comes to harbour both adults and larval forms. Since infection passes from one host to another by eating tissue infected with larvae, the life cycle in man comes to a halt. Among carnivorous animals, infection can be passed on to another animal. Man is infected by eating undercooked, trichinosed pork meat. Pigs get infected by eating infected rats or when fed on uncooked infected pork.

Trichinosis may be a serious and fatal disease. It is characterized by severe gastrointestinal disturbances, fever, pneumonitis and muscular pains. The diagnosis is difficult. Marked eosinophilia is suggestive. The worms are difficult to recover from feces, as also, the larvae in blood during the migration period. During this period precipitation and complement fixation test and skin test (using a saline extract of larvae as the antigen) are employed. Later the diagnosis can be confirmed by demonstrating encysted larvae in muscle (deltoid, gastrocnemius, and biceps.

LABORATORY DIAGNOSIS:

The laboratory diagnosis of infection by the intestinal nematodes consists of examination of feces for ova or larvae. The specimen of stool should preferably be collected after a salt purgative. It may be necessary to employ one of the concentration methods. Zinc sulphate centrifugal floatation method is one of the best methods both for ova and cysts.

DEMONSTRATIONS:

1. An adult hookworm: Note the size, brown colour and the bent anterior end. The size is comparable to that of Threadworm and differentiation is by the brown colour.
2. Mouth parts of *Ancylostoma duodenale* showing two pairs of plates.
3. An ovum of hookworm (*Necator americanus* or *Ancylostoma duodenale*) colorless, oval (60 μ × 40 μ) and segmented with a clear space between it and the eggshell.
4. Adult male female of *Ascaris lumbricoides*: The male is smaller and with a curved posterior end.
5. A fertilized egg of *Ascaris lumbricoides*: Round or oval, 60 μ × 40 μ and unsegmented. There are coarse yolk granules, a thick colorless eggshell and a thick mamillated albuminous coat stained brown due to exposure to bile.
6. An unfertilized ovum of *A. lumbricoides*: It is longer but narrower than the fertilized egg (size-90 μ × 55 μ). It has a thin egg shell, an irregular albuminous coat and contains numerous, highly refractile yolk granules.
7. Adult *Trichuris trichiura*: Note the slender anterior portion and the thicker posterior portion.
8. An ovum of *T. trichiura*: It is barrel shaped (50 μ × 20 μ) with prominent poles (which appear as mucous plugs); the ovum is unsegmented and the outer eggshell is brown.
9. Adult *E. vermicularis*; 60 μ × 30 μ. It is plano-convex, one side being definitely flatter than the other. There is a formed larva inside the colorless eggshell.
10. Stained muscle showing an encysted larva of *T. spiralis*.
11. *S. stercoralis* larva in stool.

.PRACTICAL AND EXERCISE:

1. Examine the given specimen of feces and identify the ova/cyst. Draw a diagram of the findings.

2. Concentration techniques of stool

Mouth parts of hookworms- *A. duodenale*

***A. duodenale* - Ovum**

***A. Lumbricoides* -adults-male & female**

***A. lumbricoides* - Ovum**

***T. trichiura* -Adult worm**

***T. trichiura* - Ovum**

***E. vermicularis* -female**

***E. vermicularis* - Ovum**

***T. spiralis* - encysted larva in muscle**

Larva of *S. stercoralis*

Date:________________

PRACTICAL-40

NEMATHELMINTHES: TISSUE NEMATODES

The group of tissue nematodes includes worms known as filariae and the worm *Dracunculus medinensis* (guinea worm).

A) FILARIAE:

Filariae are long and slender. The female is viviparous (has larvae and not eggs). The larvae (called microfilariae) are liberated in the tissues and find their way to blood vessels (except in the case of *O. volvulus*). The microfilariae of different worms vary in size. They are actively motile. Microfilariae (*W. bancrofti* and *B. malayi*) are found in peripheral blood at night and microfilariae (*L. loa*) during the day; the other microfilariae exhibit no periodicity.

The life cycle is passed in two hosts. The intermediate host is either a mosquito or a biting-fly. In the body of the mosquito or the fly, the microfilariae undergo metamorphosis into infective forms, but multiplication does not occur. The infective larvae migrating to the mouthparts of the insect are deposited in the definitive host. The larvae take a few months to a few years to mature into adult worms.

HABITAT:

Wuchereria bancrofti and *Brugia malayi*	- lymphatics.
Onchocerca volvulus and *Loa loa*	- subcutaneous tissues.
Acanthoceilonema perstans and	- subserous tissues of abdomen and
Mansonella azardi	- thorax

The diagnosis chiefly rests on the demonstration of microfilariae in blood and other sites. Wet coverslip preparations and stained thin and dehaemoglobinized, thick smears are examined. In the wet preparation their large size and active movement easily detect the microfilariae. For species-diagnosis a stained smear is necessary. A skin test with antigen derived from dog heart worm (*Dirofilaria immitis*) is also employed. The antigen is only group specific. The adult parasite or microfilariae can be seen in sections of tissues. Four common filariae are considered here.

1. **Wuchereria bancrofti (Lymphatic filariasis):** The infection (filariasis) is common in tropics and subtropics. It is common in our country, particularly along the seacoast. The vector is *Culex* and other mosquitoes (*Aedes* and *Anopheles*).

The males and females are found coiled up in the lymphatics and measure 4cm × 0.1 mm and 10 cm × 0.3 mm respectively. Lymphangitis, varicosity of lymphatics and collection of lymph due to rupture of the latter at various sites result in chylothorax, chylous ascites, chyluria etc. blockage of the lymphatics following recurrent attacks of lymphangitis lead to 'elephantiasis' of extremities, scrotum, penis, etc.

The microfilariae are found in chylous fluid and, at night in peripheral blood. They measure 300 μ × 10 μ and are sheathed. The column of nuclei does not reach the tip of the tail.

2. **Brugia malayi (Lymphatic filariasis):** The adults resemble those of *W. bancrofti* and the clinical disease is identical. The microfilariae are however, different. Nuclei extend up to the tip with small discrete gap between the last two nuclei. It shows many secondary curves and kinks.

3. ***Loa loa* (eye worm):** Adults are migratory and found in subcutaneous and sometimes subconjunctival tissues. Transient, painless swelling appears on the body (Calibar swellings).

B. *Dracunculus medinensis:*The definitive' host is man and intermediate host is a crustacean-Cyclops.

The adults live in the viscera or deep somatic tissues. The male is much smaller than the female and is short - lived. The gravid female (measuring about a meter), at the end of its natural life span, migrates to the subcutaneous tissues. A blister forms on the skin which ruptures and larvae are discharged from the prolapsing end of the worm when the affected part comes in contact with water. The intermediate host (Cyclops) ingests the larvae. Man is infected by drinking water containing the infected Cyclops. The subcutaneous lesion appears after long symptomless incubation (9 months to 1 year).

The diagnosis becomes self-evident when the cutaneous lesion develops. Larvae can be obtained by washing the affected part in cold water. They measure 500-750 μ × 15-25 μ and are characterized by long, tapering tails and watch-spring like movement.

DEMONSTRATIONS:

1. A stained smear of the peripheral blood showing larva of *W. bancrofti*. Note the sheath and nuclei reaching the tip.
2. A stained smear of the peripheral blood showing *B. malayi*: Note the sheath, a nucleus at its tip and another a little proximal to it.
3. An adult female of *D. medinensis*: Note the length of about 1-meter.
4. A larva of *D. medinensis* a long tapering tail.
5. A Cyclops.

PRACTICAL AND EXERCISE:

PBS showing microfilariae

Tail tips of microfilariae

Larva of *D. medinensis*

Cyclops

EXTRA SPACE

Date:________________

PRACTICAL-41

MEDICAL ENTOMOLOGY

The Medical Entomology is that branch of Zoology, which deals with the study of insects of bio-medical importance. A brief account of them is necessary to appraise their importance in relation to transmission of disease, as they affect human hosts in the following ways:

- They act as 'biological vectors' of the disease.
- Pathogenic organisms may undergo cyclical development and multiplication in insect, e.g. malarial parasite in mosquito or simply multiplication e.g. *Y. pestis* in rat fleas.
- House flies act as mechanical vectors to carry organisms like *V. cholerae*, by their soiled feet.
- They invade skin and produce skin lesions, e.g. *Sarcoptes scabei* (itch mite)
- Insects are often pests to man as they produce lesion by mechanical trauma, e.g. bite of bed bug and then lesions are secondarily infected.
- Bed bugs are also suspected to act as vectors in the transmission of Hepatitis B.

PHYLUM ARTHROPODA:

Characteristics: Invertebrates, symmetrical segmented body, exoskeleton, appendages, and sexes differentiated.

- Insect (hexopoda) e.g. Tick, Mite,
- Crustacea, e.g. Cyclops,
- Chilopoda,
- Diplopoda.

Key to medically important insects:

1) One pair of wings and straight proboscis - Dipthera (Files, Mosquitoes).
2) Body laterally compressed, no wings - Siphonoptera (Fleas)
3) Body flattened dorsoventrally, no wings - Anoptera (Lice)
4) Proboscis jointed, flexed, ventrally placed, two pairs of wings - Hemiptera (True bugs).

INSECTS OF MEDICAL IMPORTANCE:

Sr. No.	Name of insects	Diagnostic morphology	Disease related (to be filled by students)
1.	*Anopheles* mosquito	Palpi as long as proboscis, breed in clear water, lay solitary eggs, larvae lie parallel to water surface	
2.	*Culex* mosquito	Breed in polluted water, eggs in larvae lie angular to water surface	
3.	*Aedes* (House mosquito)	Silvery scales on body	
4.	Sandflies (Phlebotomous)	Wings raised over body (45° C) when at rest, body and wings covered with hairs, palpai longer than head	
5.	Deerflies (Chrysops)	Conspicuous marking on wing	
6.	*Musca domestica* (House fly)	Breed in dirty places, egg larva maggot pupa-fly	
7.	Tsetse fly (glossina)	Honey brown fly, with bayonet-like proboscis	
8.	Human flea	Wingless insects flattened laterally 3 long pairs of legs	
9.	Stable fly (*Stomoxys alcitrons*)	Blood sucking fly resembling house fly	
10.	*Xenopsylla cheopis* (Rat flea)	Ocular bristle in front of eye, rest as other fleas	
11.	Lice (*Pediculus humanis*)	Wingless, dorsoventrally flattened 3 pairs of legs claws in their terminal ends	
12.	Bed bugs (*Climas lectularic*)	Flattened body flexed Proboscis	
13.	Triatoma panatrengylus megistus (Bugs)	Segmented proboscis elongated head, wings present	

INSECTS OF MEDICAL IMPORTANCE:

Sr. No.	Insect	Diagnostic features	Disease related (to be filled by students)
1.	Hard Tick (Dermacenter)	Flattened dorsoventrally 4 pairs of legs dorsal shield, mouth parts seen dorsally	
2.	Soft tick (Orhithodorus)	No dorsal shield mouth pairs seen ventrally, similar to bed bugs.	
3.	*Sarcopies scabei* (Itch mite)	Oval, flattened, 4 pairs of legs, front leg with suckers in both sexes	
4.	Tramincula mite	5 pairs of legs, body covered with hairs	

Mosquito- Female *Culex*

Female – *Anopheles*

Body Louse

Tick

Mite

Rat Flea

Sand Fly

Self Directed Learning

1. Draw a Life Cycle of *E. histolytica*

2. Draw a Life Cycle of *Giardia lamblia*

3. Draw a Life Cycle of *Plasmodium*

4. Draw a Life Cycle of *Leishmania donovani*

5. Draw a Life Cycle of *Taenia*

6. Draw a Life Cycle of *E. granulosus*

7. Draw a Life Cycle of Schistosomes

8. Draw a Life Cycle of *Ascaris lumbricoides*

9. Draw a Life Cycle of *Ancylostoma duodenale*

10. Draw a Life Cycle of *Trichuris trichiura*

11. Draw a Life Cycle of *E. vermicularis*

12. Draw a Life Cycle of *Strongyloides stercoralis*

13. Draw a Life Cycle of *Wuchereria bancrofti*

14. Draw a Life Cycle of *Dracunculus medinensis*

EXTRA SPACE